やさしい
メディカル英語

Medical English

髙木久代 編著

講談社

編著者

高木久代　鈴鹿医療科学大学 保健衛生学部 教授（6〜9章）

著者

小澤淑子　鈴鹿医療科学大学 看護学部 教授（1〜5, 10章）

西牟田祐美子　人間環境大学 看護学部 准教授（11〜13章）

医学的内容原案・監修

東 英一　鈴鹿医療科学大学 医用工学部 教授（1, 2, 13章）

豊田長康　鈴鹿医療科学大学 学長（6〜8章）

二井英二　鈴鹿医療科学大学 保健衛生学部 教授（9, 10, 12章）

西村 甲　鈴鹿医療科学大学 保健衛生学部 教授（11章）

矢田 公　鈴鹿医療科学大学 教授（3〜5章）

英文監修

Theresa Kannenberg　修文大学 看護学部 非常勤講師（全章）

はじめに

私たち人間は，加齢とともに身体が弱り，色々な病気や怪我にみまわれることから逃れることはできません。今日，日本では高齢化が進み高齢者の割合は世界一であるといわれています。医療分野においては，高齢化に伴う疾患の複雑化により高度な医療の必要性とともに，患者の体の一部分を治療するのではなく，体全体を治療するホリスティック（holistic）な治療が重要になっています。これらの状況から，医療は各分野の専門家たちがともに患者を治療する「チーム医療」へと変わってきました。この「チーム医療」を支えるすべての医療分野の専門家（医師，看護師，薬剤師，放射線技師，理学療法士，臨床検査技師，臨床工学技士，管理栄養士，鍼灸師，他）には高度で幅広い医療知識が求められています。本書は医療を専攻する学生が一年次から英語で「解剖学」「疾患」を学習することに焦点を当てた教材です。医療を専攻する学生にとって，身体を系統的に学ぶ「解剖学」，各臓器に関わる「疾患」の学習は不可欠です。一年次から医療に不可欠かつ基礎的な知識を英語と日本語で学ぶことにより，理解を深めることができるとともに，英語を専攻しない学生にとっては英語を学習する動機づけにもなると思います。さらに，将来医療の専門職で使える特殊な英語語彙・表現を学ぶことにより，在学中のみならず卒業後も医学論文により高度な医療知識を取得するための英語力を習得していただくことを目的としています。本書を活用することで，英語力のさらなる向上がなされることを願っております。

最後に，本書を出版することができましたのは講談社サイエンティフィクの三浦洋一郎様をはじめ，皆様のご支援によるところが大きく，心より感謝申し上げます。

2018年6月　著者一同

【本書の特長】

1. 13章からなり，人体について幅広い内容と疾患について学習します。
2. 各章の【Medical Terminology〈医療専門語彙〉】，【Medical Reading〈医療英文・解剖学・疾患〉】を学ぶことにより，解剖生理学，疾患，英語論文読解，医療カルテの理解に役立てることができます。
3. 各章の【Medical Dialog】は解剖生理学，疾患理解に関連した会話内容ですので，会話を通して疾患を理解することができます。
4. 各章にある【Grammar Review〈文法の復習〉】は医療分野の論文や記事の理解に必要な英文法です。よく復習し理解するようにしましょう。
5. 本書は医学分野への編入学や大学院進学の受験勉強にも使用していただくことを念頭に置き作成しています。

Contents

Chapter

1 Cells and DNA

細胞とDNA

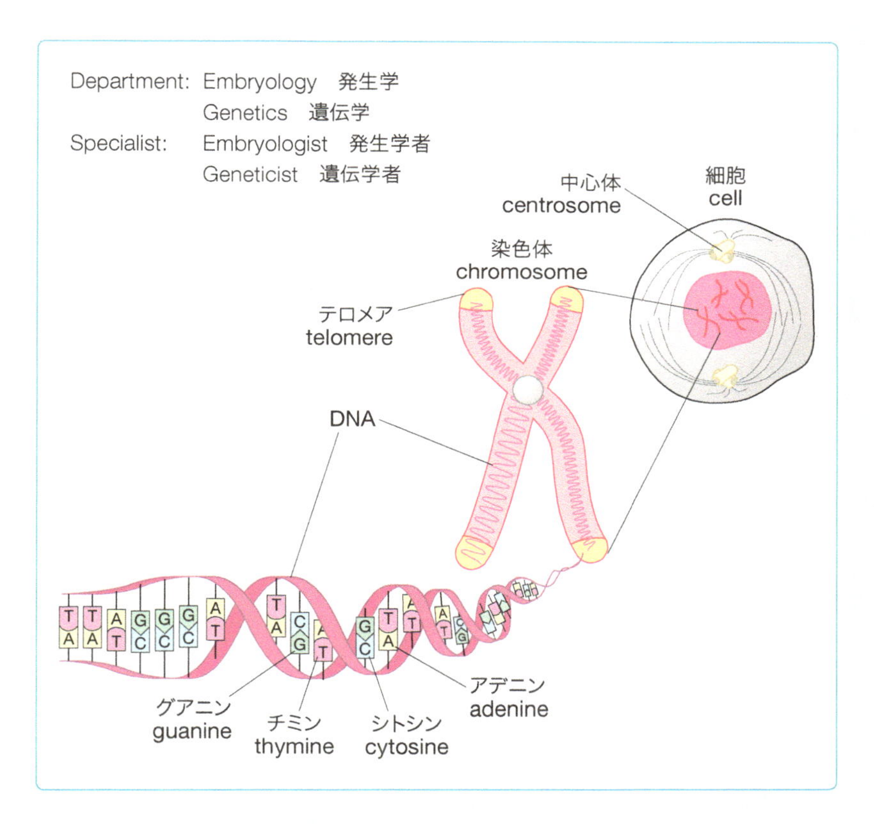

Objectives of this Chapter 本章の目的

Anatomy and physiology	Understanding the cell and DNA 細胞とDNAの理解
Disease	Learning pathology of cancer and microbiome がんとマイクロバイオームの学習
Dialog	Discussing cancer relevant to microbes がんに関連のある微生物についての対話
Grammar review	Reviewing sentence patterns 1·2 文型1·2の復習

Anatomy and Physiology of Cells and DNA

細胞とDNAの解剖生理

Medical Terminology

genetic information	遺伝情報
deoxyribonucleic acid	デオキシリボ核酸（DNA）
cytoplasm	細胞質
cell membrane	細胞膜
cytosol	細胞質基質
organelle	細胞小器官
ribosome	リボソーム
mitochondrion	ミトコンドリア（mitochondriaは複数形）
nucleus	核
double helix	二重らせん
ion	イオン
potassium	カリウム
amino acid	アミノ酸
glucose	ブドウ糖
gene	遺伝子
chromosome	染色体
DNA molecule	DNA分子
replication	複製
cell division	細胞分裂

Find answers to the following questions. 質問の答えを読み取ろう。

Q1. What is the entity of genetic information?

Q2. In what is the cytoplasm enclosed?

Q3. What organelle is relevant to energy generation?

Q4. What organelle functions to make protein?

Q5. What is included within the nucleus?

Q6. What is the structure of DNA?

Q7. How many pairs of chromosomes does a human have?

Q8. What is allocated into two cells equally by replication through cell division?

Like father, like son. This is because genetic information is conveyed from parents to children. The entity of genetic information is called deoxyribonucleic acid (DNA). Where is the DNA and how is it constructed? To gain the answers of these questions, let's learn the smallest unit of an organism, a cell which is composed of cytoplasm enclosed by a cell membrane.

The cytoplasm is filled with cytosol and organelles such as nucleus, ribosome and mitochondria. Cytosol contains resolved ions such as potassium, proteins, amino acid, glucose etc. The nucleus preserves the double helix structured DNA which includes genes and the information inside them. Chromosomes are visible in the nucleus during certain phases of cell division. The genetic information is carried out to ribosome in the cytoplasm where protein is synthesized based on the information. Mitochondria play an important part of making energy.

A human body has 46 chromosomes, in 23 pairs, half of which are inherited from his/her father and the other half from his/her mother. A chromosome is a series of DNA molecules. DNA is allocated into two cells equally by replication through cell division. Completing accurate replications of chromosomes is indispensable in conveying correct genetic information to the next generation.

Exercise Fill in the blanks with English. 空所に適する語句を英語で答えなさい。

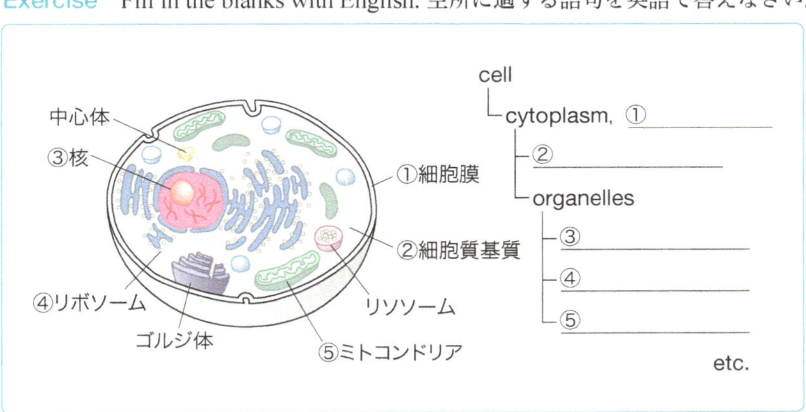

Cancer and Microbiome

がんとマイクロバイオーム

Medical Terminology

adenocarcinoma	腺がん
antibiotic	抗生物質
anticancer	抗がん性の
antivirus	抗ウイルス薬
bacterium	細菌（複数形はbacteria）
Barrett esophagus	バレット食道
butyric acid	酪酸
cancer	がん
coexist	共生する
DNA insult	DNA傷害
enteric bacterium	腸内細菌
esophagitis	食道炎
free radical	フリーラジカル，遊離基
fungus	菌類
gastric acid	胃酸
gastritis	胃炎
gut	消化管，腸，胃
Helicobacter pylori	ヘリコバクター・ピロリ
immune	免疫の
infection	感染
intestinal bacterial flora	腸内フローラ
metabolic product	代謝産物
microbe	微生物
microbiome	マイクロバイオーム
pathogenic	病原性の
vaccination	予防接種
virus	ウイルス

Find answers to the following questions. 質問の答えを読み取ろう。

Q1. What is the microbiome?

Q2. What are included in microbes besides bacteria?

Q3. How many kinds of microbes does a person have?

Q4. What do microbes to develop cancer?

Q5. How can we prevent some microbe infections?

Q6. How can we cure some microbe infections?

Q7. How do enteric bacteria spread to other parts of the body?

Q8. How do some microbes show anticancer effect?

Q9. What can *Helicobacter pylori* cause in the stomach?

Microbiome is microbes which live in the human body. Enteric bacteria or intestinal bacterial flora are some of the well-known microbiomes. Microbes include bacteria, viruses, and funguses. It is however, only a handful kinds that are pathogenic for the body. A person has more than 1,000 kinds of microbes and the gross weight is no less than 1.5kg. Most of these microbes have no influence but co-exist within the human body.

Microbes can affect cancer preventively or disadvantageously. In fact, they are obvious causes of cancer in 15-20% cases. They induce DNA insult and generate metabolic products including free radicals. Moreover, they influence functions of a person's immune cells. So, their infections are generally recommended to be prevented by vaccinations or cured by antibiotics or antiviruses.

Effects by enteric bacteria do not stay only in the gut. They can enter the blood stream with their metabolic products and immune cells to reach all over the body through the liver and may cause cancer. Some microbes, however, show an anticancer effect by producing butyric acid. *Helicobacter pylori* may cause gastritis and/or stomach cancer, called adenocarcinoma. Whereas, pH in the stomach is lowered by *Helicobacter pylori*, which reduces gastric acid resulting in restraint of Barrett esophagus and esophagitis (adenocarcinoma). Thus, microbiome controls cancer development.

Useful information マイクロバイオーム

本文にあった1.5 kgを超えるマイクロバイオームは，人間の体内に残るために淘汰されたものと言えます。それ以外のマイクロバイオームやその死骸は，水分（便の約80％），食物残渣（食物の残りカス），消化器官の細胞の剥がれたものと共に便の一部として排泄されます。

Dialog about Microbes Relevant to Cancer

がんに関連する微生物についての対話

Match the English with each Japanese term. 次の語句と英語表現を結びなさい。

肝がん	・	・	epipharyngeal cancer
子宮頸がん	・	・	hepatoma
上咽頭がん	・	・	penile cancer
陰茎がん	・	・	cervical cancer

Find the English in the dialog for the following Japanese. 次の日本語を表す英語を対話文中から抜き出しなさい。

B型，C型肝炎ウイルス　（　　　　　　　　）

ヒトパピローマウイルス　（　　　　　　　　）

エプスタイン・バールウイルス　（　　　　　　　　）

注）infectious mononucleosis：伝染性単核症，kissing disease（キス病）は俗称

Useful information さまざまな腫瘍

腫瘍（tumor）は悪性（malignant）の腫瘍と良性（benign）の腫瘍に区別されますが，一般に，がんとよばれるのは悪性の腫瘍です。がんの名称を「～がん」と表すとき，英語では“... cancer”といったり“cancer of ...”といったりします。その他にも非常に多くの種類の腫瘍があるので，ほんの一部ですが紹介します。

白血病	leukemia（血液のがん，2章参照）
リンパ腫	lymphoma（白血球の中のリンパ球の腫瘍）
肉腫	sarcoma（骨や脂肪，筋肉，神経などから発生）
脳腫瘍	brain tumor（頭蓋内のあらゆる組織から発生）
黒色腫	melanoma（皮膚，眼窩内組織，口腔粘膜上皮などに発生）

Student (S): I learned that some microbes are relevant to cancer but I don't know which microbes cause cancer.

Teacher (T): Don't you know about hepatitis B and C viruses?

S: I know about them. As the name implies, they develop hepatitis not cancer.

T: Hepatitis B and C are caused by viruses and if patients are not treated, some patients develop hepatoma.

S: That's awful. I remember hearing some news about a vaccination for cancer of the uterine cervix. What is the name of that virus?

T: It is human papillomavirus. The virus causes both cervical cancer and penile cancer.

S: Really? I haven't heard of penile cancer before.

T: Moreover, malignant lymphoma and epipharyngeal cancer may be caused by the Epstein-Barr virus or EB virus.

S: Oh, it's the virus of kissing disease, isn't it?

T: Do you know the formal name for the kissing disease?

S: I have no idea. What is it called in the medical field?

T: It is called infectious mononucleosis.

S: I should remember the name.

T: Yes, you should. EB virus causes not only the infectious mononucleosis but also malignant lymphoma or epipharyngeal cancer.

S: Sounds serious.

Exercise　Indicate if these are true (T) or false (F). 対話文の内容に合っている（T）か，合っていない（F）か答えなさい。

1. Hepatitis B and C are cancer caused by viruses.
2. There is no vaccination for cancer.
3. EB virus may cause penile cancer.
4. The kissing disease is another name for infectious mononucleosis.

Grammar Review 文型(1·2)

第1文型　日本語の主語・述語にあたるものを英語では主語subject（S）・動詞（または述語動詞）verb（V）といいます。基本的な文では最初にくる「〜は，〜が」という文の中心になる語が主語，主に主語の動きを表すのが動詞です。次のように主語（S）と動詞（V）だけでも文ができますし，それに修飾語modifier（M）をつけて長い文を作ることもできます。

Birds fly.
S V
鳥は 飛ぶ。

Birds fly high in the sky.
S V M
鳥は空高く飛ぶ。

He walks.
S V
彼は 歩く。

He walks with his wife in the park every morning.
S V M
彼は毎朝妻と公園を歩く。

このようにSVの文を第1文型といいます。Mがあっても第1文型です。

第2文型　それでは，第2文型はどのようなものかというと，SVに補語complement（C）が加えられます。補語はSVだけでは，文として正確な意味が表せない場合に意味を補う役割をし，次のようにSと同じものを表します（S = C）。この第2文型の動詞にはbe動詞がよく使われますが，知覚を表すfeel, look, soundなど，状態を表すkeep, seem, stayなど，変化を表すget, become, growなども使われます。

She is a nurse. she = a nurse
S V C
彼女は看護師だ。

She is a nurse in the US.
S V C M
彼女は米国で看護師をしている。

They looked happy. They = happy
S V C
彼らは幸せそうに見えた。

They looked happy during the party.
S V C M
彼らはパーティーの間幸せそうに見えた。

Exercise　Answer "S, V, C, M" and the meaning of each sentence. 次の文の要素（S，V，C，M）を示し，意味を答えなさい。

1. She smiled.
2. He got old.
3. She smiled at the baby.
4. He got old after retiring at the age of 65.

Chapter 2

Blood

血液

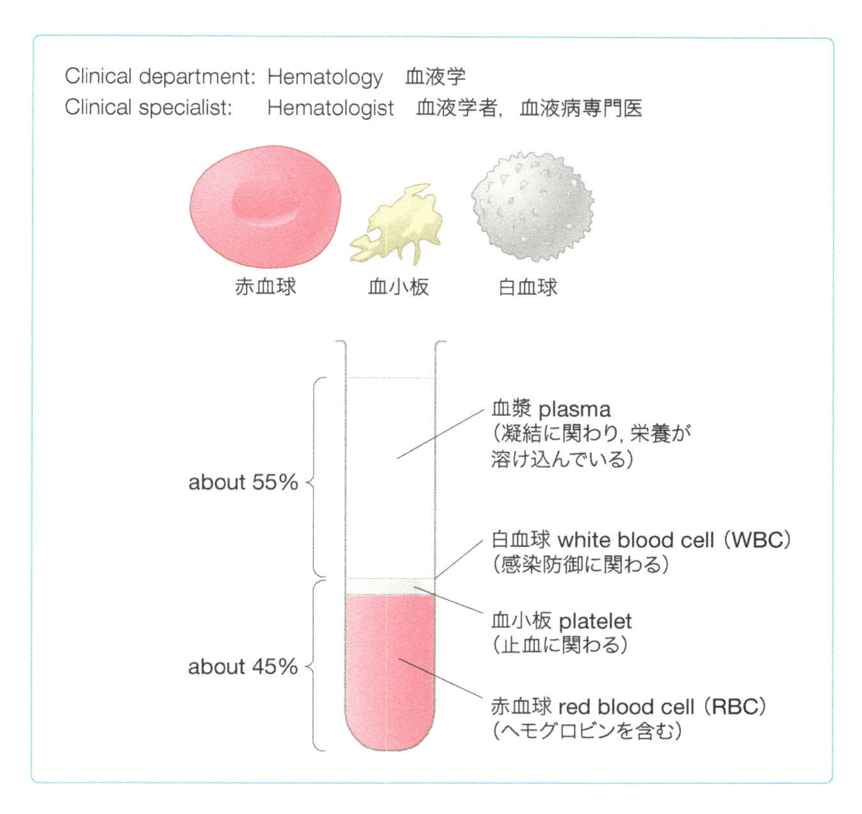

Objectives of this Chapter 本章の目的

Anatomy and physiology	Understanding the functions and the constituents of blood 血液の機能と組成の理解
Disease	Learning pathology of leukemia and how it was discovered 白血病とその発見についての学習
Dialog	Discussing prefixes, suffixes etc. concerning blood 血液に関する接頭辞・接尾辞などについての対話
Grammar review	Reviewing sentence patterns 3·4·5 文型3·4·5の復習

Anatomy and Physiology of Blood

血液の解剖生理

Medical Terminology

acquired immunity	獲得免疫
ADP (adenosine diphosphate)	アデノシンニリン酸
blood vessel	血管
bone marrow	骨髄
coagulation	凝固
coagulation factor	凝固因子
erythrocyte	赤血球
hematopoietic stem cell	造血幹細胞
hemoglobin	ヘモグロビン
intestine	腸
leukocyte	白血球
lymphocyte	リンパ球
monocyte	単球
natural immunity	自然免疫
neutrophil	好中球
nutrient	栄養素
oxygenation	酸素化
phagocytosis	食作用
plasma	血漿
platelet	血小板
red blood cell (RBC)	赤血球
secrete	分泌する
venous blood	静脈血
white blood cell (WBC)	白血球

Find answers to the following questions. 質問の答えを読み取ろう。

Q1. What is the yellowish liquid called?

Q2. What percentage of blood is a red solid?

Q3. What turns red by oxygenation?

Q4. Why is the color of WBCs unnoticeable in blood?

Q5. What increases during the natural immunity process?

Q6. What is acquired immunity strengthened by?

Q7. What blood cells are largest in number?

Q8. What stops the bleeding in the body?

When blood in a test tube is left to stand for an hour, it divides into a red solid and a yellowish liquid. Measuring the two components, the red solid containing blood cells is about 45% and the yellowish liquid called plasma is approximately 55% of the entire blood volume in the test tube. The red solid is made from red blood cells also known as erythrocytes or RBCs, surrounded by white film-like white blood cells also called leukocytes or WBCs, and the platelets. Blood cells are derived from hematopoietic stem cells in the bone marrow.

The RBCs, the main component of blood cells, contain hemoglobin. Hemoglobin transports oxygen from the lungs to the body tissues and iron in the hemoglobin turns the RBCs red through oxygenation. Venous blood looks dark red when it finally returns to the heart after its journey through the human body.

The white color of the WBCs is generally not noticeable in blood because the number of WBCs is about 1/500 of that of RBCs. One of the methods of protecting the body from infection is to increase WBCs (neutrophils and monocytes), which have the function of phagocytosis, an important defense against infection. After WBCs are produced in and released from bone marrow, they increase in number within several hours. Neutrophils increase first and monocytes increase later. This process, natural immunity, is effective as a primary reaction against bacteria, whereas lymphocytes respond quickly to secondary infections. This process is called acquired immunity and can be strengthened by vaccinations.

The platelets are also white and their number is 1/25 of that of RBCs. Their function is connected to the process of blood coagulation. Platelets gather around the damaged site of the blood vessel and then various substances are released around the site to begin the blood coagulation process. The stuck platelets secrete ADP, by which the platelets along with other coagulation factors become sticky and thus the bleeding stops.

Plasma includes various nutrients which are received from the intestines and delivered to all parts of the body.

Leukemia

白血病

Medical Terminology

acute	急性の	fatigue	疲労，倦怠
acute transformation	急性転化	imatinib	イマチニブ
basophil	好塩基球	leukemia	白血病
bone marrow aspiration	骨髄穿刺	lymphocytic	リンパ系の
bruising	皮下出血斑	myelogenous	骨髄性の
chemotherapeutic	化学療法薬	night sweat	寝汗
chromosome abnormality	染色体異常	Philadelphia chromosome	フィラデルフィア染色体
chronic	慢性の	poor appetite	食欲不振
diagnose	診断する	therapeutic	治療の
donor	ドナー	translocate	(染色体を)転移させる
dosage	投薬量	transplantation	移植
enzyme	酵素	tyrosine kinase	チロシンキナーゼ
eosinophil	好酸球		

Find answers to the following questions. 質問の答えを読み取ろう。

Q1. What becomes cancerous?

Q2. What causes lack of normal cells?

Q3. What type of leukemia is composed of immature cells?

Q4. What type of leukemia grows slowly?

Q5. What is the Philadelphia chromosome?

Q6. What do drugs such as imatinib inhibit?

Q7. What are the symptoms of chronic myelogenous leukemia?

Q8.Why do patients look pale and show bruising?

Q9. What is an expected cure for leukemia?

Q10. How can leukemia be detected?

Leukemia is cancer of the leucocytes or immature leucocytes, which are normally part of the body's defense system. WBCs develop from hematopoietic stem cells in bone marrow. When some cells develop abnormally, meaning some parts of the chromosomes change, it is called chromosome abnormality resulting in abnormal cell division. The forever increasing number of chromosomes with abnormality become cancerous resulting in leukemia. The high number of leukemia cells in the bone marrow then suppress the development of normal cells such as neutrophil, basophil, eosinophil and monocyte.

There are four types of leukemia: acute lymphocytic, acute myelogenous, chronic lymphocytic and chronic myelogenous. Acute leukemia, which is composed of immature cells, progresses rapidly whereas chronic leukemia, which is constituted of comparatively mature cells, progresses slowly.

In cases of chronic myelogenous leukemia, two specific translocated chromosomes called Philadelphia chromosomes create abnormal enzymes called tyrosine kinase and cause a disorder in the growth pattern of WBCs. Medicine like imatinib is administered in order to inhibit tyrosine kinase.

Patients with acute transformation associated with chronic myelogenous leukemia suffer from fatigue, poor appetite, weight loss, fever and night sweats. They look pale with bruising caused by the lack of normal blood cells and may only live a few months if left untreated.

A cure for leukemia is expected in some cases through combining a high dosage of chemotherapeutics with transplantation of hematopoietic stem cells when the patient has a proper donor, a supplier of hematopoietic stem cells. The four different types of leukemia can be detected and diagnosed during a physical examination, with a blood sample test and/or a bone marrow aspiration which can show the abnormal increase in WBCs leading to proper treatment.

Dialog about Blood

血液についての対話

Match the English with each Japanese term. 英語と意味を結びなさい。

pathologist	・	・	細胞遺伝学者
cytogeneticist	・	・	病理学者
suffix	・	・	接頭辞
prefix	・	・	接尾辞
anemia	・	・	貧血
uremia	・	・	尿毒症

Pick up words with the following prefixes and suffixes from the dialog. 次の接頭辞と接尾辞を含む語を対話文から抜き出しなさい。

leuk- または leuc- ( )

erythro- ( )

-emia ( )

-cyte ( )

Teacher (T): Do you know the prefix leuk- or leuc-?

Student (S): No. But I learned the words leukemia and leucocyte.

T: That's right. Leukemia is made of leuk- and -emia.

S: The dictionary says leuk- means white. Is leukemia white?

T: The quantity of leucocyte is usually small so we can't see the color. But a German pathologist named Rudolf Virchow observed many leukemia cells in a patient's blood.

S: Many leucocytes looked white, didn't they?

T: Yes, good for you! Then what does -emia mean?

S: May I consult the dictionary?

T: Yes, using a dictionary is very helpful to learn languages. But before that, can you remember some other word with -emia?

S: Let me see. Uremia has -emia on the end. Oh, I know another word with -emia, anemia. Does -emia indicate blood disease?

T: Yes. You should also check -cyte of leucocyte and erythrocyte as well as erythro-.

S: OK. I found that -cyte means cell.

T: Yes.

S: And well, erythro means red. It's exciting to check prefixes and suffixes.

T: A dictionary has a lot of information. So make use of it!

S: I will. But may I ask one thing?

T: Go ahead. Asking questions is also important.

S: Does the name Philadelphia chromosome have anything to do with the city in the US?

T: Yes. A cytogeneticist in the city of Philadelphia, USA discovered the chromosome abnormality of cancer.

Exercise Indicate if these are true (T) or false (F). 対話文の内容に合っている（T）か，合っていない（F）か答えなさい。

1. The prefix leuk- means red.
2. The suffix -emia shows color.
3. Dictionaries show suffixes.
4. Virchow is a city in Germany.
5. The philadelphia chromosome is named after the city in the US.

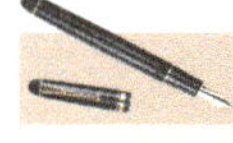

Useful information Rudolf Virchow

ドイツの病理学者。日本ではウィルヒョウ，フィルヒョー，ヴィルヒョーなどとして知られている。静脈血栓症の形成に関する三つの要因（血管の障害・血流の鬱滞・血液性状の変化）は彼の名を付けて「ウィルヒョウの三徴」と呼ばれている。また，胃がんが左鎖骨上窩に転移することは，ウィルヒョウ転移として広く知られている。

Grammar Review 文型(3·4·5)

第3文型SVO　目的語object（O）は動詞Vの目的・対象となる語で，「〜を」という意味になります。意味がSVCではS＝CであるのにSVOではS≠Oであるのも見分けるコツです。

He drank sake.
S　V　O
彼は酒を飲んだ。

He drank sake for the first time in Japan.
S　V　O　M
彼は日本で初めて酒を飲んだ。

第4文型SVOO　2つのOを間接目的語indirect object（IO），直接目的語direct object（DO）と表すこともあります。IOは「〜に」，DOは「〜を」の意味を表します。

She showed me a book.
S　V　O　O
彼女は私に本を見せてくれた。

She showed me a book last week.
S　V　O　O　M
彼女は先週私に本を見せてくれた。

第5文型SVOC　この文型のCはOの補語で，O＝Cとなります。Oは「〜を」，Cは「〜と」と訳せます。

We called him Boss.
S　V　O　C
我々は彼をボスと呼んだ。

We called him Boss for his leadership.
S　V　O　C　M
我々は彼の統率力のため彼をボスと呼んだ。

Exercise　Answer "S, V, O, C, M" and write the meaning of each sentence. 次の文の要素（S，V，O，C，M）を示し，意味を答えなさい。

1. We study English.
2. I gave her a bag.
3. The movie made me happy.
4. We study English to understand other people in the world.
5. I gave her a bag as a birthday present yesterday.
6. The movie made me happy from the beginning.

Chapter 3

The Cardiovascular System

心臓血管系

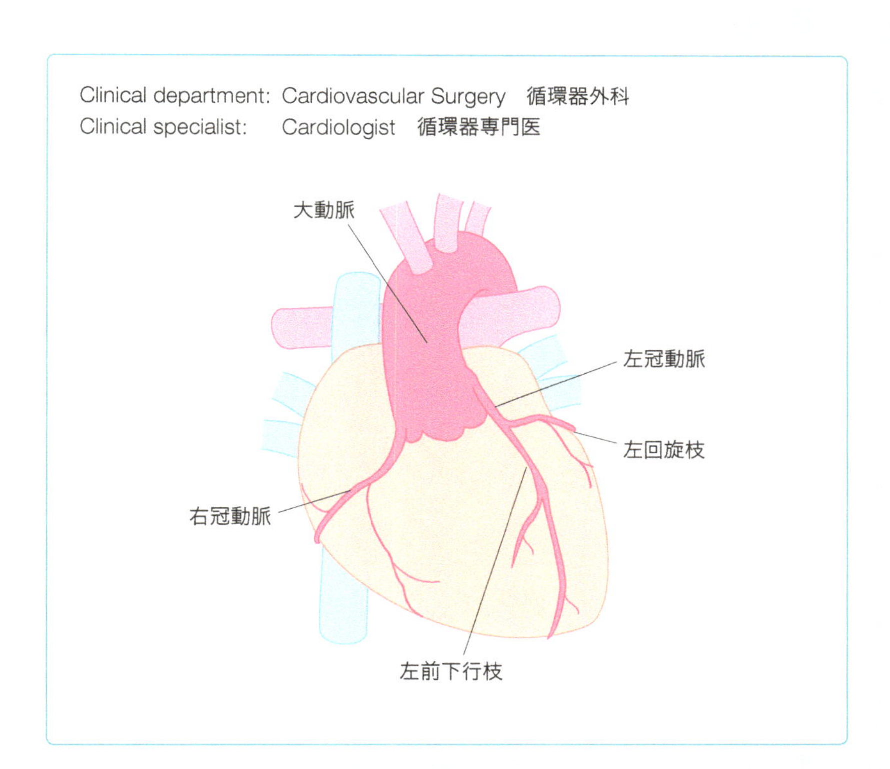

Objectives of this Chapter　本章の目的

Anatomy and physiology	Understanding the structure and functions of the heart and blood vessels 心臓と血管の構造と機能の理解
Disease	Learning pathology of ischemic heart disease 虚血性心疾患についての学習
Dialog	Discussing the valves of the heart 心臓の弁の名称，形状などについての対話
Grammar review	Reviewing noun usage 名詞の復習

Anatomy and Physiology of the Cardiovascular System

心臓血管系の解剖生理

Medical Terminology

aorta	大動脈	gas exchange	ガス交換
arterial blood	動脈血	heart beat	心拍
atrioventricular node	房室結節	inferior vena cava	下大静脈
atrium	心房（atriaは複数形）	mediastinum	縦郭
bundle of His	ヒス束	myocardium	心筋層
cardiac muscle	心筋	pacemaker	歩調とり
cardiovascular system	心臓血管系	pulmonary artery	肺動脈
conducting system	刺激伝導系	pulmonary vein	肺静脈
contraction	収縮	Purkinje fiber	プルキンエ線維
coronary artery	冠状動脈	sinoatrial node	洞房結節（洞結節）
diastole	拡張期	superior vena cava	上大静脈
electric irritability	電気的興奮	systole	収縮期
electrocardiography	心電図検査（ECG）	ventricle	心室
endocardium	心内膜	ventricular septum	心室中隔
epicardium	心外膜		

Find answers to the following questions. 質問の答えを読み取ろう。

Q1. What does the cardiovascular system consist of?

Q2. Where is the heart?

Q3. Where does the venous blood flow just before the right ventricle?

Q4. What flows out through the pulmonary veins to the aorta?

Q5. What are the two phases of the heart beat?

Q6. Where does the stimulation of the conducting system of the heart start?

Q7. What arteries supply blood to the heart?

The cardiovascular system consists of the heart and blood vessels. The heart is located in the mediastinum in the center of the chest. Constituted of two atria and two ventricles, the heart is the size of an adult fist and weighs approximately 300g. The wall of the heart has three layers: the endocardium, myocardium and epicardium.

The venous blood, which comes from the upper body into the superior vena cava and from the lower body into the inferior vena cava, flows into the right atrium and flows out through the pulmonary artery from the right ventricle. Blood flows into the lungs and undergoes gas exchange becoming arterial blood. The arterial blood flows into the left atrium through four pulmonary veins and then is pumped out from the left ventricle through the aorta to the entire body. Generated by the contraction of the cardiac muscle, the heart beat is controlled by the pacemaker called the conducting system of the heart. Stimulation of the conducting system of the heart starts from the sinoatrial node near the opening for the superior vena cava of the right atrium. It reaches the Purkinje fiber, which is divided into right and left bundles, through the atrioventricular node near the ventricular septum and bundle of His. The heart beat has two phases called systole and diastole whose electric irritability can be recorded by an electrocardiography (ECG).

Five percent of blood is supplied to the heart. The right coronary artery which feeds the right and bottom part of the heart, while the left coronary artery is responsible for the left part. (cf. p.17)

Exercise Fill in the blanks with English. 空所に英語で名称を記入しなさい。

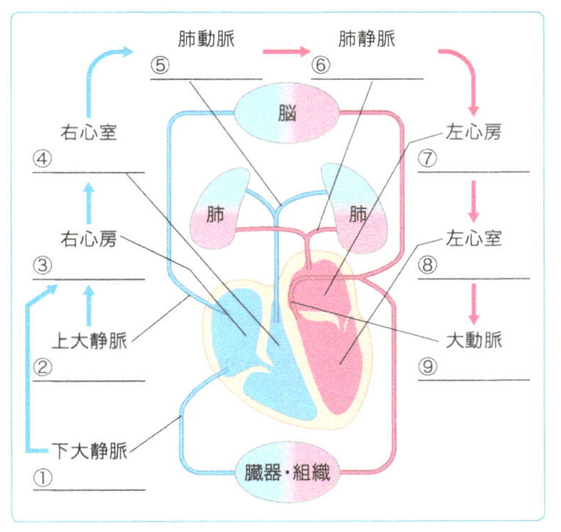

Ischemic Heart Disease

虚血性心疾患

Medical Terminology

angina pectoris	狭心症
anterior	前方
arrhythmia	不整脈
arterial lumen	動脈内腔
arteriosclerosis	動脈硬化
atheroma	アテローム
cardiac catheterization	心臓カテーテル検査
cardiac rehabilitation	心臓リハビリテーション
coronary artery bypass grafting	冠動脈バイパス術（CABG）
coronary CT	冠動脈CT
diabetes	糖尿病
echocardiography	心エコー検査
heart failure	心不全
hyperlipidemia	高脂血症
hypertension	高血圧
ischemia	虚血
ischemic heart disease	虚血性心疾患
mortality rate	死亡率
myocardial infarction	心筋梗塞
necrosis	壊死
nuclear medicine scan	核医学検査
obesity	肥満
occlusion	閉塞
oppression	圧迫感
percutaneous coronary intervention	経皮的冠動脈形成術（PCI）
pharmacotherapy	薬物療法
rupture of the heart	心破裂
stable angina	労作性狭心症
stenosis	狭窄
thrombosis	血栓症
tightness	絞扼感
transient	一過性の
unstable angina	不安定狭心症

Find answers to the following questions. 質問の答えを読み取ろう。

Q1. What are the risk factors of arteriosclerosis?

Q2. How is ischemic heart disease classified?

Q3. What is the main symptom of angina pectoris?

Q4. What is a myocardial infarction caused by?

Q5. How is ischemic heart disease diagnosed?

Q6. What treatment is effective for some angina pectoris?

Ischemic heart disease, also known as coronary artery disease, is a condition that affects the blood and oxygen supply to the heart due to narrowed or blocked heart arteries. Risk factors associated with arteriosclerosis are hyperlipidemia, hypertension, diabetes, obesity, smoking and/or family medical history. This disease is classified into two groups according to the narrowing degree of the arterial lumen: angina pectoris and myocardial infarction.

Angina pectoris is caused by transient ischemia and the main symptom is chest pain characterized by a feeling of chest tightness or oppression in the left anterior part that spreads to the left shoulder and arm. It is identified at the time it occurs: Stable angina occurs during times of physical activity, and unstable angina occurs during periods of rest.

Myocardial infarction is the condition of necrosis caused by a coronary artery disorder by severe stenosis or complete occlusion by thrombosis from atheroma. It leads to severe arrhythmia, heart failure, shock, rupture of the heart etc., and the mortality rate is as high as 30%.

Ischemic heart disease is diagnosed through blood sample test, electrocardiography (ECG), nuclear medicine scan, echocardiography, coronary CT and cardiac catheterization. Pharmacotherapy, percutaneous coronary intervention (PCI) or coronary artery bypass grafting are effective for some angina pectoris patients. Treatment for arrhythmia, heart failure or shock as well as cardiac rehabilitation is necessary for myocardial infarction, however, full recovery of heart function cannot be achieved.

Exercise　Fill in the blanks. 空所に適語を記入しなさい。

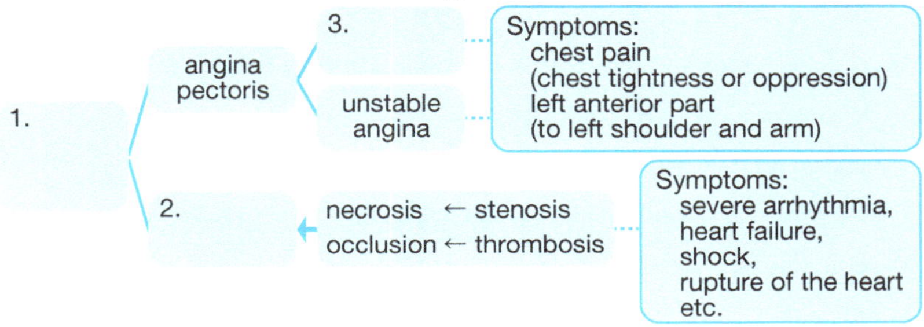

Dialog about Valves

弁膜についての対話

Match the English with each Japanese term. 英語と意味を結びなさい.

aortic valve	・	・	三尖弁
pulmonary valve	・	・	肺動脈弁
tricuspid valve	・	・	大動脈弁
mitral valve	・	・	僧帽弁

Student A: Have you learned the names of the four valves?

Student B: Not really. It is easy to remember the aortic valve and pulmonary valve.

A: I agree. The aortic valve is the valve toward the aorta, and the pulmonary valve is the valve toward the pulmonary artery.

B: Yes. And their shapes are similar, too.

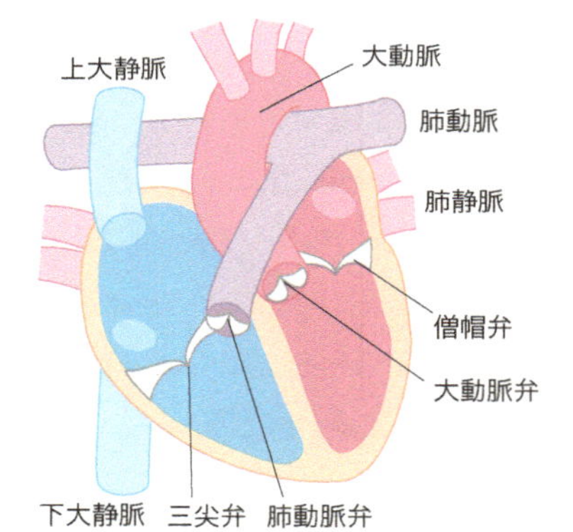

A: These two are valves between the ventricles and arteries.

B: And the rest are between the atrium and ventricles.

A: The valve between the right atria and right ventricle is …

B: The tricuspid valve.

A: Yes. It has three cuspid-like pieces which open and close.

B: Tri means three and we can imagine there are three pieces in the valve.

A: Do you know what a cuspid is?

B: I checked my dictionary. A cuspid means a dogtooth.

A: Good for you! Does the piece of the tricuspid valve look like a dogtooth?

B: I don't know. I can see my dogteeth but I've never seen the actual valve.

A: Me neither. I can't imagine the whole shape of the valve piece from just the picture of the valve.

B: Since the name was chosen, it must really look like it.

A: OK. The fourth valve is the mitral valve.

B: I've heard it is also named after a shape of a mitral. First of all, I don't know what a mitral is. Do you know what it is?

A: I searched for it on the Internet. Here is a picture of a mitral.

B: Oh, I've seen a Catholic bishop wearing this on TV. It is easier to imagine the leaves of the valve.

A: I think so, too. The valve is between the left atria and left ventricle.

B: Now I can remember the names of the four valves!

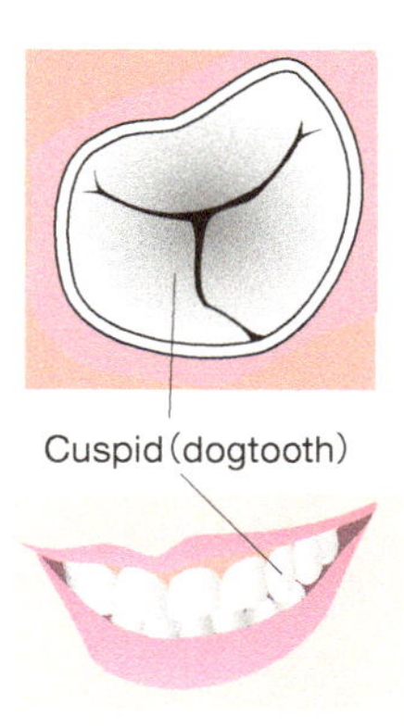

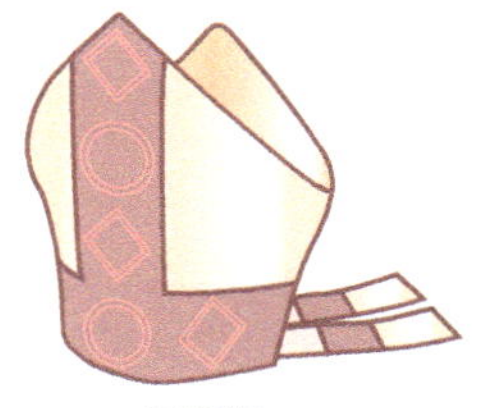

司祭帽

Exercise Indicate if these are true (T) or false (F). 対話文の内容に合っている（T）か，合っていないか（F）か答えなさい。

1. The name of aortic valve suggests where it is.
2. The pulmonary valve is in the lungs.
3. The tricuspid valve has three cuspid-like pieces.
4. Shapes of the mitral valve and pulmonary valve are similar.

Exercise Fill in the blanks with the valve names. 適切な弁の名称を記入しなさい。

Valves in English and Japanese	Position
1.	Between the left ventricle and the aorta
2.	Between the right ventricle and the pulmonary artery
3.	Between the right ventricle and right atria
4.	Between the left ventricle and left atria

Grammar Review 名詞(nouns)

名詞は，文の要素としては主語，目的語，補語として使われます（その他，修飾語としても使われます）。

The scientists named the element Nihonium.

S	V	O	C
科学者（名詞）		元素（名詞）	ニホニウム（名詞）

また，名詞には次のような種類があります。

可算名詞　countable noun　机，木，家族，人々など数えられる名詞

普通名詞　common noun　e.g.）a book, books　数えられ，複数形がある

集合名詞　collective noun　全体で見れば単数扱い，個々を見れば複数扱い

e.g.）The staff is capable.　The staff are all kind.

e.g.）His family lives in Mie.　My family are all tall.

不可算名詞　uncountable noun　数えられない名詞

固有名詞　proper noun　e.g.）Japan, Mt. Fuji　複数にせず単数扱い

物質名詞　material noun　e.g.）blood, oxygen　形が不定で単数扱い

抽象名詞　abstract noun　e.g.）peace, knowledge　抽象的概念で単数扱い

Exercise 1　Label the S, V, O, C and M of each sentence and underline the nouns.
各文の要素S，V，O，C，Mを示し，名詞に下線を引きなさい。

1. His classmate checked the dictionary.
2. The arterial blood gives the cells nutrients.
3. The heart is a muscle organ.
4. Pathologists call the condition arrhythmia.

Exercise 2　Choose the correct form of each noun. 適切な形の名詞を選びなさい。

1. The (doctor/ doctors) always manages the patient's (condition/ conditions).
2. The (patient/ patients) suffers from various (symptom/ symptoms).
3. (People/ Peoples) in the lab discovered a new (bacteria/ bacterium).

Chapter

4 Respiratory System

呼吸器系

Clinical department: Respiratory Medicine 呼吸器内科
Clinical specialist: Pulmonologist 呼吸科医

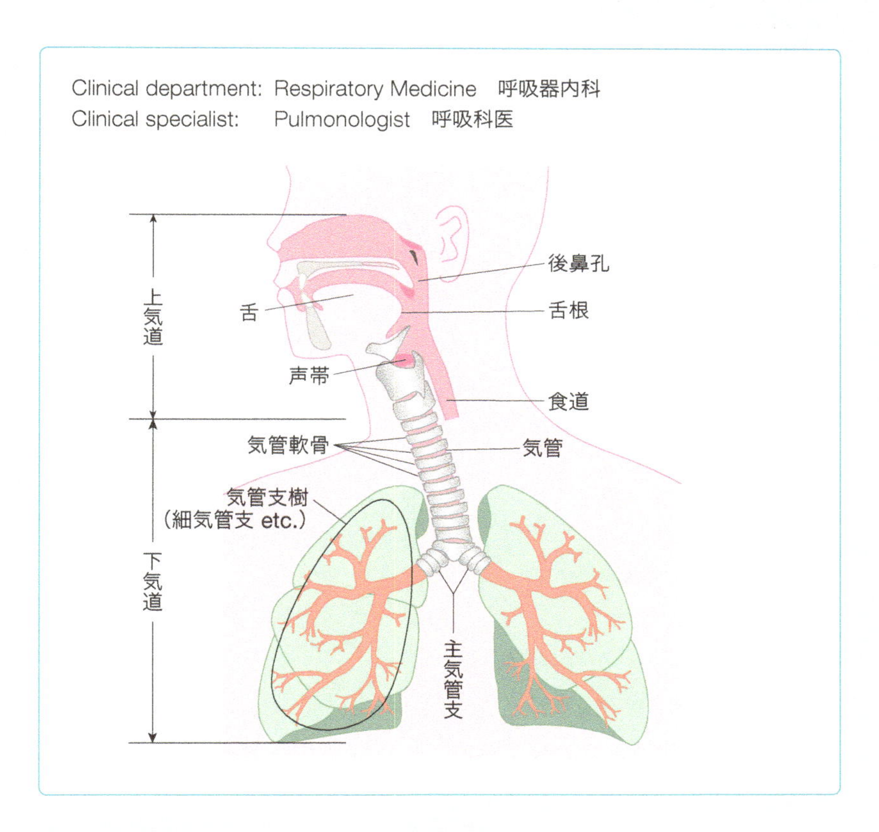

Objectives of this Chapter 本章の目的

Anatomy and physiology	Understanding the functions and the constituents of the pulmonary system 呼吸器系の機能と構成の理解
Disease	Learning pathology of Chronic Obstructive Pulmonary Disease 慢性閉塞性呼吸器疾患の病理の学習
Dialog	Discussing the alveoli 肺胞についての対話
Grammar review	Reviewing functions of adverbs 副詞の働きを復習する

Anatomy and Physiology of the Respiratory System

呼吸器系の解剖生理

Medical Terminology

airway	気道	lower airway	下気道
alveolus	肺胞(複数形はalveoli)	nerve	神経
bronchial tree	気管支樹	nerve cell	神経細胞
bronchiole	細気管支	pharynx	咽頭
bronchus	気管支(複数形はbronchi)	pleura	胸膜(複数形はpleurae)
choana	後鼻孔	primary bronchus	主気管支
ciliary movement	線毛運動	respiratory	呼吸の
cough reflex	咳嗽反射	root of tongue	舌根
esophagus	食道	sputum	痰
filtrate	濾過する	superior nasal concha	上鼻甲介
foreign body	異物	thoracic vertebra	胸椎
gas exchange	ガス交換	trachea	気管
humidification	加湿	tracheal cartilage	気管軟骨
larynx	喉頭	upper airway	上気道
lobe	(上葉, 中葉, 下葉などの)葉	vocal cord	声帯

Find answers to the following questions. 質問の答えを読み取ろう。

Q1. What composes the lower airway?

Q2. How many lobes does the right lung have?

Q3. How thick is the trachea?

Q4. Where does the trachea branch into the bronchi?

Q5. Which angle is more acute to the trachea, the right or left bronchus?

Q6. How does a coughing occur?

Q7. How does sputum eliminate microbes or dust?

Q8. Where are sounds produced?

The respiratory system composed of the lungs and airway is responsible for taking in oxygen and releasing carbon dioxide with the muscles of respiration. Covered with pleurae, the right lung has three lobes while the left lung has only two. The airway is divided into the upper airway which is composed of the nose, mouth, pharynx and larynx, and the lower airway which includes trachea, bronchi and bronchioles.

The pharynx is from the choanae to the esophagus and the larynx is between the root of the tongue and trachea. The trachea is 10 to 15 cm long, 2.0 to 2.5 cm in diameter and has a series of 15 to 20 U-shaped tracheal cartilages in front of the esophagus. It branches into right and left primary bronchi at the height of the fifth thoracic vertebra behind the heart. The right bronchus is 2.5 cm long and turns at an angle of 25° to the trachea whereas the left one is 5 cm and at 35°. The bronchi enter the lungs together with vessels and nerves. Each bronchus continues to branch off more than 23 times until it reaches the alveoli in the interior of the lungs. These are called bronchial trees and serve to deliver air to the more than 300 million tiny alveoli.

Besides the primary function of gas exchange, the respiratory organs have many important functions: coughing expels foreign objects by cough reflex against chemical or physical stimuli in the pharynx, larynx, trachea or primary bronchi; ciliary movement eliminates microbes or dust as sputum in the trachea; and others such as warming and humidification of air, smelling by the nerve cells in the superior nasal concha, controlling the movement of food or air in the pharynx and producing sounds by the vocal cords in the larynx.

Exercise Draw an illustration of the respiratory system including ① larynx, ② trachea, ③ right and left bronchi and ④ right and left lungs. ①喉頭，②気管，③左右の気管支，④左右の肺を含む呼吸器系のイラストを描きなさい。

Chronic Obstructive Pulmonary Disease (COPD)

慢性閉塞性肺疾患

Medical Terminology

allergen	アレルゲン	inflammatory	炎症性の
allergy	アレルギー	inhale	吸う，吸い込む
attack	発作，発病	irreversible	不可逆性の
bronchial asthma	気管支喘息	obstructive	閉塞性の
bronchiectasis	気管支拡張症	pathogen	病原体
bronchitis	気管支炎	pneumonia	肺炎
chronic obstructive pulmonary disease	慢性閉塞性肺疾患，COPD	progressively	進行性に
diffuse panbronchiolitis	びまん性汎細気管支炎	quality of life (QOL)	生活の質
exertional dyspnea	労作時呼吸困難	respiratory rehabilitation	呼吸リハビリテーション
home oxygen therapy	在宅酸素療法 (HOT)	WHO (World Health Organization)	世界保健機関

Find answers to the following questions. 質問の答えを読み取ろう。

Q1. What are lungs exposed to while they perform their functions?

Q2. What kind of disease is COPD?

Q3. What causes COPD?

Q4. What percentage of COPD patients had smoked at least once according to 2004 WHO survey?

Q5. What is the ninth highest cause of death in 2010 in Japan?

Q6. How is COPD distinguished from bronchial asthma?

Q7. What is necessary for patients with COPD?

Q8. What is provided for serious patients of COPD to help improve QOL?

The lungs, while performing their function, are exposed to various pathogens and dust particles, which may lead to serious lung diseases such as bronchitis, pneumonia or lung cancer. In addition to these diseases, we should know another disease chronic obstructive pulmonary disease (COPD).

COPD is an inflammatory and irreversible obstructive pulmonary disease caused by inhaling cigarette smoke and/or other harmful substances over an extended period of time. It is characterized by gradual development of exertional dyspnea, chronic coughs and sputum with advancing age. Ninety percent of patients with COPD have a history of smoking, and the disease was the fourth highest cause of death in the world in 2004 according to the WHO survey. In Japan, it was the ninth highest cause of death in 2010, and presently, 8.6% of Japanese who are 40 years of age or older have the disease.

It is necessary to differentiate COPD from bronchial asthma, diffuse panbronchiolitis or bronchiectasis. COPD and bronchial asthma especially need careful discrimination. The former develops progressively in adults over the age of 40 and the chronic symptoms cannot be completely relieved even with treatment, whereas the latter disease often develops in younger people with attacks caused by physical exercise, emotional episodes, allergic reactions to dust or other allergens, and the symptoms can be relieved with treatment.

Patients with COPD should be prohibited from smoking, given respiratory rehabilitation as well as appropriate pharmacotherapy. Moreover, home oxygen therapy (HOT) is provided for serious patients in order to improve quality of life (QOL). WHO is presently promoting the prohibition of smoking worldwide in order to decrease the number of new cases of COPD.

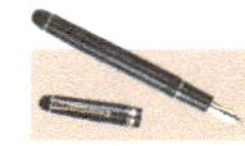

Useful information 健康日本21

わが国では生活習慣病の予防を目的とした「健康増進法」を平成25年に改正するとともに，「健康日本21（第2次）」を制定し，がん，循環器疾患，糖尿病およびCOPDの予防・早期発見などの対策がなされてきている。

Dialog about Alveoli

肺胞についての対話

Match the corresponding vocabulary. 正しい読み方を選びない。

m^2	・	・	micrometer
μm	・	・	square meter
10^{-6}	・	・	a hundred million
100,000,000	・	・	ten to the power of minus six

Fill in the blanks with words in the dialog. 対話文から抜き出して書きなさい。

meaning	singular form	plural form
肺胞	alveolus	①
気管支	②	bronchi
半径	radius	③
刺激	④	stimuli

meaning	singular form	plural form
細菌	bacterium	⑤
卵子	⑥	ova
データ	datum	⑦
媒体	⑧	media

Teacher (T): Today you've learned that the gas exchange is performed on the surface of the many alveoli.

Student (S): Wait, do you mean the word alveoli is in the plural form?

T: Yes, it is. I think you've heard the singular form of alveoli, haven't you?

S: Is it alveolus?

T: That's right. The plural form of some words such as bronchus, radius and stimulus, ends with -i. That is, bronchi, radii, stimuli are the plural forms.

S: That's interesting. We've learned that the plural forms of bacterium, ovum, datum and medium are bacteria, ova, data and media.

T: Great! You've learned a lot. These words are derived from Latin.

S: Oh, Latin still remains in our lives although it is said to be a dead language.

T: Most languages interact with each other.

S: I see. I enjoyed sidetracking. Shall I get back to discussing the alveoli?

T: Sure. Do you have any questions?

S: Yeah. How large is each alveolus?

T: Each one is about 250-300 μm in diameter.

S: Micrometer? Micro means ten to the power of minus six, doesn't it?

T: Yes. That's correct, the diameter of each alveolus is 0.25-0.30 mm.

S: Smaller than 1 mm!

T: Gas exchange occurs through diffusion between the surface of alveoli and the capillary plexus.

S: Capillary plexus covers every alveolus and gas exchange occurs there.

T: That's right. It occurs through diffusion between the surface of alveoli and the capillary plexus.

S: Diffusion. That is, when the oxygen rate is higher in the alveoli than in the capillaries, oxygen moves to the capillaries. And when carbon dioxide is thicker in the capillaries, it diffuses into the alveoli.

T: That's a good explanation.

capillary plexus：毛細血管網

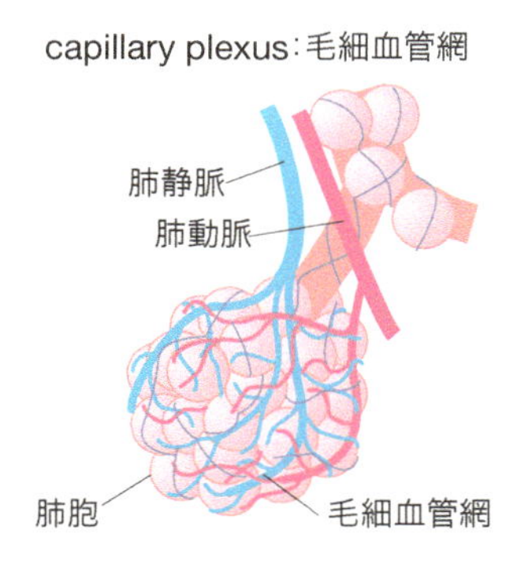

diffusion：拡散作用

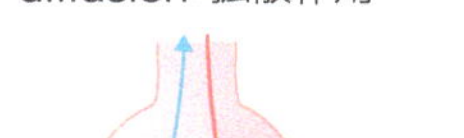

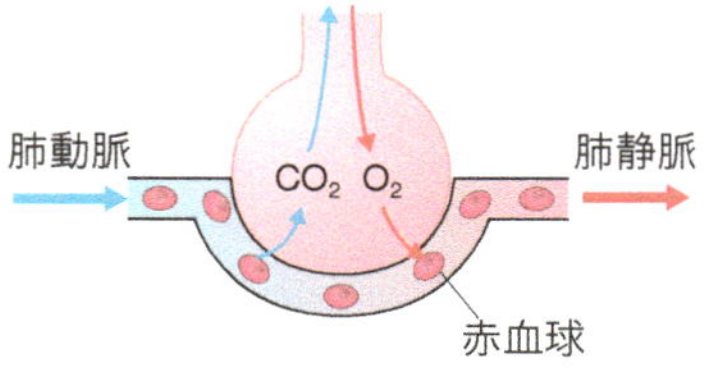

毛細血管内に多いCO_2が肺胞内に移動し，
肺胞内に多いO_2が毛細血管内に移動する。

Exercise Indicate if these are true (T) or false (F). 対話文の内容に合っている（T）か，合っていない（F）か答えなさい。

1. The plural ending “i” comes from Latin.
2. The weight of each alveolus is 250-300 micrograms.
3. The diameter of an alveolus is not as large as 1mm.
4. Diffusion functions for gas exchange in the lung.

Grammar Review 副詞(adverb)

副詞 副詞が修飾するのは通常，動詞，形容詞，他の副詞，句，節，文全体です。形容詞と間違えやすいので注意しよう（形容詞については次章）。

verb adverb The family lived happily.	副詞 動詞 その家族は幸せに暮らした。
adverb adjective His idea is completely new.	副詞 形容詞 彼の考えは完全に新しい。
adverb adverb She drew quite beautifully.	副詞 副詞 彼女はきわめて美しく描いた。
adverb sentence Finally he passed the test.	副詞 文 ついに彼はその試験に合格した。

頻度を表す副詞（always, usually, often, sometimes, rarely, seldom, never等）
一般動詞の前，be動詞・助動詞の後ろに置きます。

I can always help him.	私はいつも彼を助けることができる。
He usually walks carefully.	彼はたいてい注意深く歩く。
She is sometimes busy in summer.	彼女は夏には時々忙しい。
They seldom go out at night.	彼らはめったに夜，外出しない。

Exercise Double underline the adverbs, underline the modified words and put each sentence into Japanese. 副詞に二重下線，副詞が修飾している語に下線を引き，和訳しなさい。

1. He ate a very large pie.
2. She is singing cheerfully.
3. They told us the way kindly.
4. Luckily, they could understand the language.

Chapter 5

The Digestive System

消化器系

Clinical department: Gastroenterology 消化器科
Clinical specialist: Gastroenterology physician 消化器内科医

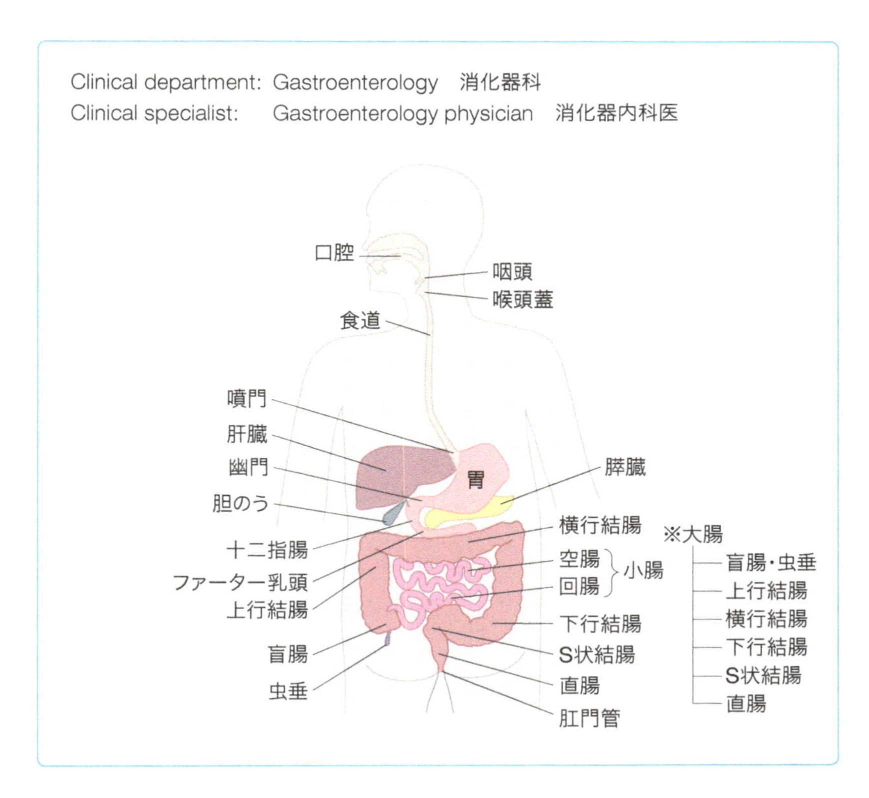

Objectives of this Chapter 本章の目的

Anatomy and physiology	Understanding the functions and the constituents of the Digestive System 消化器系の機能と構成の理解
Disease	Learning pathology of liver disease 肝臓疾患の病理の学習
Dialog	Discussing the islet of Langerhans ランゲルハンス島についての対話
Grammar review	Reviewing functions of adjectives 形容詞の働きを復習する

Anatomy and Physiology of the Digestive System

消化器系の解剖生理

Medical Terminology

alkalescent	アルカリ性の
anus	肛門管
appendix	虫垂
ascending colon	上行結腸
aspiration	誤嚥
bile	胆汁
cardia	噴門
cecum	盲腸
descending colon	下行結腸
diaphragm	横隔膜
digestive juice	消化液
digestive system	消化器系
duodenum	十二指腸
electrolyte	電解質
endocrine gland	内分泌腺
epiglottis	喉頭蓋
exocrine gland	外分泌腺
external secretion	外分泌
gallbladder	胆嚢
gastric juice	胃液
glucagon	グルカゴン
ileum	回腸
insulin	インスリン
jejunum	空腸
Langerhans island (islet)	ランゲルハンス島
large intestine	大腸
metabolism	代謝
pancreas	膵臓
pancreatic juice	膵液
portal vein	門脈
pylorus	幽門
rectum	直腸
sigmoid colon	s状結腸
small intestine	小腸
swallowing reflex	嚥下反射
transverse colon	横行結腸
Vater's papilla	ファーター乳頭

Find answers to the following questions. 質問の答えを読み取ろう。

Q1. What prevents aspiration?

Q2. What does the Vater's papilla do?

Q3. In which blood vessel do nutrients go through to the liver?

Q4. How much digestive juice is secreted in the small intestine?

Q5. What is reabsorbed in the large intestine?

The digestive system helps the body digest food, take in nutrients and excrete waste as follows. The epiglottis in the larynx prevents aspiration through the swallowing reflex to send food to the esophagus, a 25-30 cm long tube located behind the trachea. It reaches the cardia of the stomach whose volume varies according to the food it keeps. The stomach secretes about 1,500 ml of gastric juice per day. Continuing on from the pylorus, the c-shaped duodenum has Vater's papilla, which controls the inflow of bile and pancreatic juice.

The duodenum, jejunum, and ileum constitute the small intestine, where 2,400 ml of alkalescent digestive juice promotes digestion and absorption of nutrients daily.

Nutrients are carried through the portal vein to the liver, which lies just under the diaphragm. The primary functions of the liver are metabolism, production of and external secretion of bile and its storage, and the filtration of blood. More than half of the bile from the liver is stored and recycled in the gallbladder to be reused for digestion. Near the gallbladder and behind the stomach is the pancreas which is 14-18 cm long. The exocrine glands in the pancreas secrete pancreatic juice to assist in the digestion of sugars, proteins and fats. The endocrine glands called the islets of Langerhans secrete hormones such as insulin and glucagon.

The large intestine, where water and electrolytes are reabsorbed, includes the cecum with the appendix, ascending colon, transverse colon, descending colon, sigmoid colon and rectum. The digestive system extends from the mouth all the way to the anus through which waste matter leaves the body.

Exercise　Draw an illustration of the digestive system including ①pharynx, ②esophagus, ③stomach, ④small intestine, ⑤cecum with appendix, ⑥ascending colon, ⑦transverse colon, ⑧descending colon, ⑨sigmoid colon, ⑩rectum, ⑪anus, ⑫liver, ⑬gallbladder and ⑭pancreas. ①～⑭を含む消化器系の図を描きなさい。

Hepatic Disease

肝臓疾患

Medical Terminology

alcoholism	習慣性の過度の飲酒	hepatitis A (B/C/D/E) virus	A (B/C/D/E) 型肝炎ウイルス
anticancer	抗がん（の）	hepatocellular carcinoma	肝細胞がん
autoimmune	自己免疫	inflammation	炎症
cholangiocellular carcinoma	胆管細胞がん	jaundice	黄疸
contaminate	汚染する	metabolic disorder	代謝異常
cystadenocarcinoma	嚢胞腺がん	metastatic liver cancer	転移性肝がん
fibrosis	線維化	mother-to-infant transmission	母子感染
general fatigue	全身倦怠	primary liver cancer	原発性肝がん
hepatic artery	肝動脈	prognosis	予後
hepatic cirrhosis	肝硬変	radiation	放射線
hepatitis	肝炎	terminal stage	末期

Find answers to the following questions. 質問の答えを読み取ろう。

Q1. What can be causes of acute hepatitis?

Q2. How can HBV infect the body?

Q3. What leads hepatic cells to necrosis or fibrosis?

Q4. Which virus has the highest risk of developing into hepatic cirrhosis?

Q5. What is the prospective treatment for hepatic cirrhosis?

Q6. How many people die from hepatic cirrhosis per year?

Q7. Where does metastatic liver cancer spread from?

Q8. What treatment is effective for early-stage liver cancer?

Acute hepatitis is a liver disorder caused by hepatitis viruses, drugs, alcohol etc. beginning with symptoms such as general fatigue and lack of appetite and in more serious cases jaundice. Among hepatitis viruses A, B, C, D and E, the hepatitis A virus (HAV) is transmitted through contaminated food or water. Luckily, it seldom results in chronic hepatitis. Hepatitis B and C viruses (HBV and HCV) are infected by blood and body fluids. Concerning HBV, mother-to-infant transmission is also known.

Chronic hepatitis caused by hepatitis B or C viruses, autoimmune liver diseases and metabolic disorders is inflammation of the liver that can last longer than 6 months. The hepatic cells undergo necrosis or fibrosis gradually due to prolonged inflammation and can progress to hepatic cirrhosis. Hepatitis C cases, more so than others, progress into hepatic cirrhosis.

Hepatic cirrhosis is the terminal stage of fibrosis of the liver. One of the main causes is alcoholism. There are approximately 200,000 hepatic cirrhosis patients in Japan today, and unfortunately 15,000 patients die from this disease every year. The only cure for hepatic cirrhosis is liver transplantation.

Liver cancer is classified into two groups: primary liver cancer and metastatic liver cancer. Primary liver cancer includes hepatocellular carcinoma which occurs most frequently, cholangiocellular carcinoma, cystadenocarcinoma, etc. Ninety-five percent patients of hepatocellular carcinoma are carriers of hepatitis viruses and 80% of them are HCV carriers. Metastatic cancer, which can come from the lungs, kidneys, large intestine, stomach, pancreas and other organs through the hepatic artery or portal vein, occurs 8 times more frequently than primary liver cancer. Surgical operation, radiation treatment and anticancer chemotherapy are effective for early-stage liver cancer however, liver cancer in advanced stage shows an unfavorable prognosis.

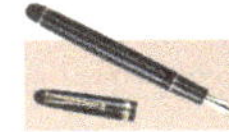

Useful information アルコール性肝硬変

アルコール性肝硬変は飲酒量と高い相関があり，アルコール換算で160 g（焼酎3～4合，日本酒で5～6合）を5年間以上にわたって長期摂取すると約80％の確率でアルコール性肝障害あるいは肝硬変になるといわれる。

Dialog about Islet of Langerhans

ランゲルハンス島についての対話

Fill in the blanks with anatomical terms relevant to scientists' names. 科学者の氏名と関係のある解剖学用語を記入しなさい。

解剖学用語	anatomical term	scientist
ランゲルハンス島		Paul Langerhans, a German pathologist
ファーター乳頭		Abraham Vater, a German anatomist
ウィリス動脈輪		Thomas Willis, an English physician
ヘンレ係蹄		Friedrich G. J. Henle, a German doctor

Fill in the blanks with diseases relevant to scientists' names. 科学者の氏名と関係のある疾患名を記入しなさい。

疾患名	disease	scientist
ファロー四徴症		Étienne-Louis A. Fallot, a French physician
クッシング病		Harvey W. Cushing, an American neurosurgeon
パーキンソン病		James Parkinson, a British physician
川崎病		Tomisaku Kawasaki, a Japanese pediatrician

Student (S): I've learned about the Langerhans islet in the pancreas. The beginning of the name is written with a capital letter. So, is this also a scientist's name?

Teacher (T): You are right. The eponym of Langerhans islet is an eponym of Paul Langerhans, a German pathologist.

S: What is an eponym?

T: An eponym is a person, place or thing after whom or which something is named. Some examples are: Vater's papilla named after Abraham Vater, a German anatomist; The circle of Willis named after an English physician, Thomas Willis; the Henle loop discovered by a German doctor, Friedrich Gustav Jakob Henle.

S: If I find a new tissue, is it possible to give it my name?

T: I think so. You can also name a disease if you find a disease. There are a lot of diseases named after their discoveries. Tetralogy of Fallot is named after a French doctor, Etienne-Louis A. Fallot, Cushing disease is after an American neurosurgeon, Harvey Williams Cushing; Parkinson's disease is from a British physician, James Parkinson; and Kawasaki disease is named after a Japanese pediatrician, Tomisaku Kawasaki.

S: Wow. By the way, is the islet of Langerhans different from the island of Langerhans?

T: Well, what do island and islet mean?

S: Both mean small land surrounded by water.

T: Yes, that's correct. They look like islands or islets among other cells: Islet or island of Langerhans, Langerhans island or islet indicate the same thing. They have cells which secrete various hormones including insulin and glucagon.

S: Yes, and if insulin is not secreted enough, then this may be a sign of diabetes.

T: That's right. In addition, you must be careful about the pronunciation and spellings of islet and island.

S: Both "s" spellings are not pronounced.

T: Are there a lot of medical terms with silent letters?

S: Well, c of muscle, b in limb, w in wrist, l in calf, k in knee, gue in tongue ...

T: Excellent! Some of others are g in benign, p in pneumonia and th in asthma.

S: I learned a lot about eponyms and silent letters from the Langerhans islet.

Exercise Indicate if these are true (T) or false (F). 対話文の内容に合っている（T）か，合っていない（F）か答えなさい。

1. Langerhans islet is different from Langerhans island.
2. Langerhans island is named after the capital city of a nation.
3. The pronunciation of island is the same as Iceland.
4. Insulin has something to do with diabetes.

Grammar Review 形容詞（adjective）

形容詞は主に名詞・代名詞を修飾したり（限定用法），文の補語になったり（叙述用法）します。品詞レベルの役割と文の要素レベルの役割があるので，注意しましょう。

限定用法の例

adjective noun
The young child stood up.

形容詞 名詞
その幼い子どもは立ち上がった。

adjective pronoun
The toy was an old one.

形容詞 代名詞
そのおもちゃは古いものだった。

通常，形容詞は名詞の前に置かれるが，次のように後ろに置かれる例もある。

pronoun adjective
He found something red.

形容詞 代名詞
彼は何か赤いもの（赤い何か）を見つけた。

叙述用法の例

S V C
The boy is brave.

主語 補語（形容詞）
その少年は勇敢である。

S V O C
He left the patient alone.

主語 目的語 補語
彼は患者を一人にしておいた。

Exercise Tell S, V, O, C and M of each sentence and underline the adjectives.
各文のS，V，O，C，Mを示し，形容詞に下線を引きなさい。

1. She holds a big doll.
2. The tall gentleman looks old.
3. A pretty woman is carrying something round.
4. I chose a new one.

Chapter 6

The Urinary System

泌尿器系

Clinical department: Urology　泌尿器科
Clinical specialist: Urologist　泌尿器専門医

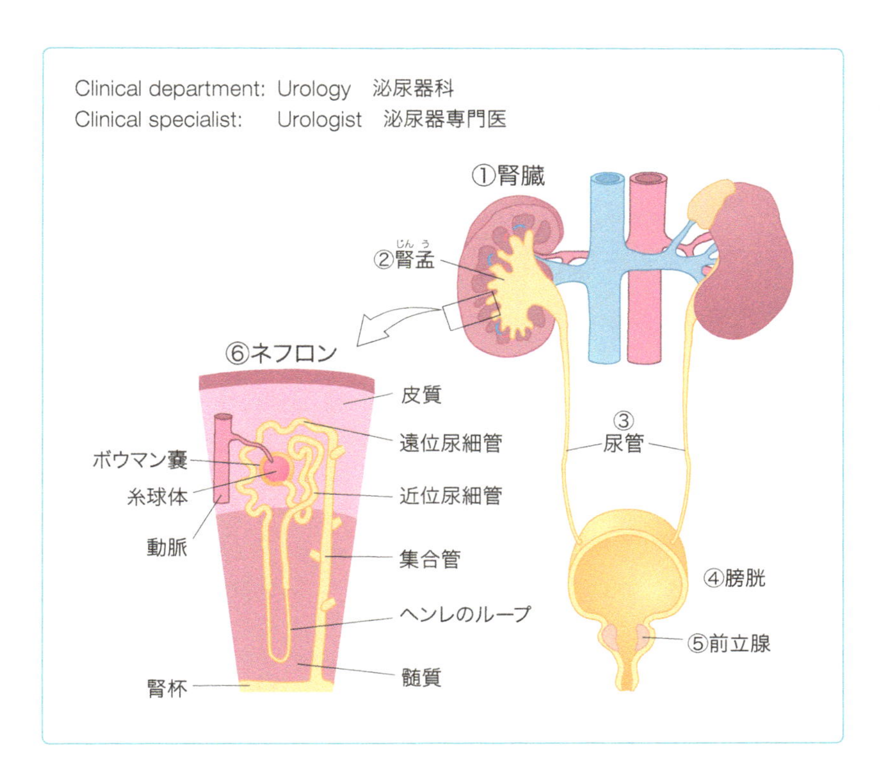

Objectives of this Chapter　本章の目的

Anatomy and physiology	Understanding functions of the urinary system 泌尿器系の機能理解
Disease	Learning about kidney stone disease 尿路結石の学習
Dialog	Discussing the symptoms of kidney stone disease and how to prevent the disease 尿路結石の症状，原因，予防について
Grammar review	Reviewing the preposition of time and place 時，場所を示す前置詞の復習

Urinary System

泌尿器系

Medical Terminology

artery	動脈	peritoneum	腹膜
bladder	膀胱	renal artery	腎動脈
Bowman's capsule	ボウマン嚢	renal cortex	腎皮質
capillary vessel	毛細血管	renal medulla	腎髄質
cluster	かたまり	renal pelvis	腎盂
elastic bag	伸縮性の袋	renal vein	腎静脈
electrolyte	電解質	ureter	尿管
glomerulus (複数形glomeruli)	糸球体	urethra	尿道
nephron	ネフロン(腎単位)	urinary track	尿路

Find answers to the following questions. 質問の答えを読み取ろう。

Q1. Where are the kidneys located?

Q2. What is urinary system composed of?

Q3. What is a nephron?

Q4. How is urine made in the body?

Q5. What are two parts of the kidney?

Q6. Where is the glomerulus?

Q7. What is the main function of the kidney?

Q8. What are the other functions of the kidney?

Q9. How long are the ureters?

Q10. How is urine excreted?

Exercise Answer the illustrations ①~⑥ in English. p.41のイラストの①~⑥の各部位を英語で書きなさい。

The urinary system is composed of two kidneys, the ureters, the bladder and the urethra. A pair of kidneys which are located on the left and right sides of the body behind the peritoneum is bean-shaped and their length is about 12 cm. The renal vein, the renal artery and nerves enter each kidney. The ways in which urine passes through are called urinary tracks, which continue from the ureter, bladder to urethra. Blood flows through thin arteries which get thinner and thinner from the renal artery and into the structure called the glomerulus that are clusters of capillary vessels. Blood finally excretes through one thick renal vein after passing from the glomerulus to the thinner vein.

Each kidney is divided into two parts: an outer region (the renal cortex) and an inner region (the renal medulla).The glomerulus is in the renal cortex and the renal tubules are in both the renal cortex and the renal medulla. The urine passing through the gathered tubules of nephron flow into the renal pelvis located in the center of the kidneys.

The smallest components of the kidneys are called nephron where blood is filtered and urine is made. Each kidney has one million nephron including Bowman's capsule, the glomeruli surrounded by the thin wall-like bowl and small renal tubules, from which urine is excreted. Urine is collected into gathered tubules from many renal tubules.

The main function of the kidneys is to keep a good balance between water and minerals including electrolytes in the body. Other functions are purifying blood, excreting the waste products produced in the body, disposing of wastes such as toxins, medicine and harmful substances, regulating blood pressure and secreting a variety of hormones. The ureter is the tubule made of muscle, 40 cm in length and its top is connected to each kidney and the bottom to the bladder. Urine produced in each kidney is sent to the bladder in small amounts by means of peristaltic movement of the ureter. The bladder is like an elastic bag made of muscle that keeps urine waste from the body.

When enough urine is gathered, a signal informing the need for urination is sent to the brain by nerves and then urine is excreted into the urethra, which is about 20 cm in length in the case of men and about 4 cm in women.

Kidney stone disease (urolithiasis)

尿路結石

Medical Terminology

blockage	閉塞
calcium stone	カルシウム結石
cystine stone	シスチン結石（含硫アミノ酸：硫黄を含むアミノ酸の一種）
endoscopic surgery	内視鏡手術
ESWL (extracorporeal shock wave lithotripsy)	衝撃波破砕術
hydronephrosis	水腎症（尿腎症）
periodically	周期的に
renal parenchyma	腎実質
struvite stone	ストラバイト結石（リン酸マグネシウムアンモニウム結石）
uric acid stone	尿酸結石

Find answers to the following questions. 質問の答えを読み取ろう。

Q1. What is a kidney stone (urolithiasis)?

Q2. What are three kinds of kidney stones?

Q3. When does the pain of kidney stone disease occur?

Q4. What disease occurs when there is a blockage of the ureter?

Q5. What are symptoms of kidney stone disease?

Q6. How is kidney stone disease diagnosed?

A kidney stone is a solid piece of material existing in the urinary system: in the renal parenchyma, renal pelvis, ureter or bladder. It originally forms in one or both kidneys and then moves to other parts of the urinary system. The size and shape of a kidney stone can vary, for example, a tiny stone must be observed through a microscope but others can be a few centimeters in diameter.

Different ingredients form different kidney stones. They include calcium stones, struvite stones, uric acid stones and cystine stones which include amino acid with sulfur.

Kidney stones may remain within the renal parenchyma or the renal pelvis. If not, they pass into the ureter or the bladder. Kidney stones may exist within the renal parenchyma or renal pelvis without pain. However if stones get stuck in the ureter while passing through severe pain will result. It is also possible for the stones to create an obstruction in the ureter and cause hydronephrosis.

The larger the stones block, the smaller the stones go through naturally. The size stones can pass is less than 5 mm in diameter. The pain is usually severe and is in the lower back or on one side of the abdomen, accompanied by vomiting, blood in the urine. The pain is unbearably severe, which occurs periodicallly and continues for 20-60 minutes.

If a large kidney stone is suspected, a CT scan can identify its location, size and severity of blockage, which can distinguish from other diseases having the same kind of pain. A urine test can show the presence of kidney stone, blood in the urine, and/or infection. Once a kidney stone has been found, its type can be identified. Doctors prescribe painkiller and medication for discharging the stones as a treatment.

If infection is present, the stone will be removed or eliminated by extracorporeal shock wave lithotripsy (ESWL) or endoscopic surgery.

Dialog about Kidney Stone Disease

尿路結石に関する対話

A: I had a severe pain when I left home two days ago. I had never experienced that kind of pain and I vomited, so I could not move at all. My mother called an ambulance and I was taken to the hospital.

B: Oh, that sounds so bad. Were you examined at the department of internal medicine?

A: Yes, Yes. The kind doctor examined me gently and gave me CT scan immediately.

B: What was the result?

A: The doctor's diagnosis was kidney stone disease. He gave me medicine which eased my pain. I was so surprised to hear I had a stone in my body.

B: Are you OK now?

A: Yes, the medicine made me much better. The doctor told me to have an operation if my pain continues. It's awful.

B: I wonder how kidney stones form in the body.

A: I read an article in a medical journal that stone forming is related to daily lives. Eating a lot of meat increase oxalic acid and uric acid in the body. These substances are usually excreted with feces. But extra oxalic acid is combined with calcium in the urine, resulting in forming a stone.

B: How can we prevent making stones in the body?

A: It is important to eat a lot of vegetables, drink a lot of water and do physical exercise every day. I must change what I do in my daily life.

B: Me too. Let's do our best to keep a healthy life.

oxtic acid：シュウ酸，uric acid：尿酸

Find answers to the following questions. 質問の答えを読み取ろう。

Q1. What are the symptoms of kidney stone disease?

Q2. How are kidney stones formed in the body?

Q3. What are prevention of kidney stones disease?

腎結石症と尿路（管）結石症　石が尿道に移行して尿路結石となる。

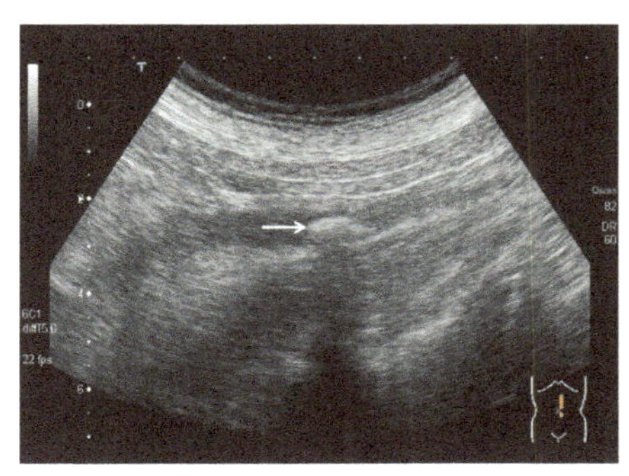

左尿管結石（超音波画像）

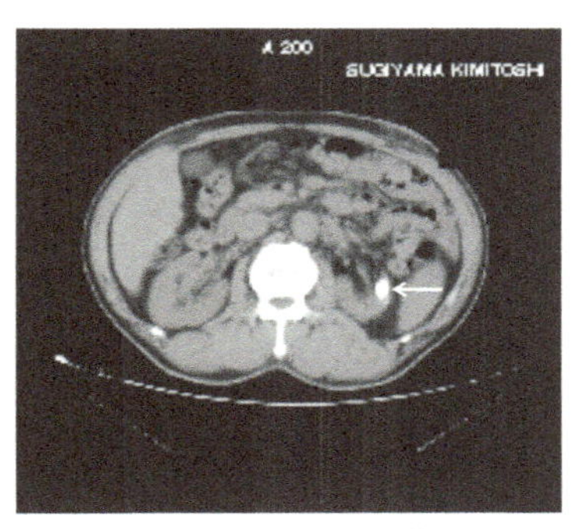

左腎結石（X線CT画像）

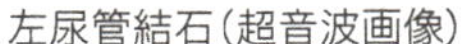

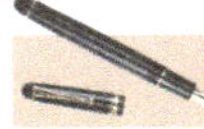

Useful information 尿路結石は食事で予防できる？

シュウ酸の摂りすぎは尿路結石の原因となります。肉類はシュウ酸を増やすため少し控え，旬の野菜を多く取るようにしましょう。また，カルシウムを多く取るようにしましょう。ただし摂りすぎてはいけません。カルシウムは小魚，牛乳，納豆，豆腐，にんじん，南瓜など緑黄色野菜に多く含まれます。水分補給も忘れずに（1日に2L以上）！

尿路結石の主な症状

わき腹周辺の激しい痛み／吐き気・冷や汗／血尿／頻尿・残尿感（結石の部位によって症状が異なる）

Grammar Review 時・場所を示す前置詞（preposition）

前置詞は名詞，名詞句の前に置きます。at, in, to, for などがあります。

「時」を示す前置詞

at：時刻，正午，真夜中
　at seven, at noon, at night, at dawn（明け方）

in：月，年，季節，午前，午後
　in April, in 2020, in summer, in the morning, in the afternoon

on：曜日，特定の日
　on Sunday, on May 5, on the weekend, on Christmas Day

※　in ～して，～をへて　after ～後に　within ～以内に

「場所」を示す前置詞

at：狭い場所で（に）　at the corner

on：接触している　on the road

below：より下のほうに
　below the bridge

under：真下に　under the table

between：～の間に
　between the building

in：広い場所で（に）　in the library

above：より上のほうに
　above the clouds

over：真上に，全面を覆って
　over the mountain

near：近くに　near the sea

Exercise　Fill in the blank. 空欄を埋めなさい。

1. I go to the library ＿＿＿＿＿ Sunday.
2. Let's meet each other ＿＿＿＿＿ 13:00 ＿＿＿＿＿ the station.
3. We can have the result of the test ＿＿＿＿＿ ten minutes.（～後に）
4. You must come back here ＿＿＿＿＿ one hour.（以内に）
5. Tom lives ＿＿＿＿＿ the park.（近くに）
6. The sun has risen ＿＿＿＿＿ the horizon.
7. We will study ＿＿＿＿＿ the library ＿＿＿＿＿ summer vacation.
8. He usually takes a walk ＿＿＿＿＿ the morning with his wife.
9. We arrived ＿＿＿＿＿ the hotel ＿＿＿＿＿ the evening.
10. They had a party ＿＿＿＿＿ June 10th.

Chapter 7

The Endocrine System

内分泌系

Clinical Department: Internal Medicine　内科

Endocrinology　内分泌科

Clinical specialist: Endocrinologist　内分泌専門医

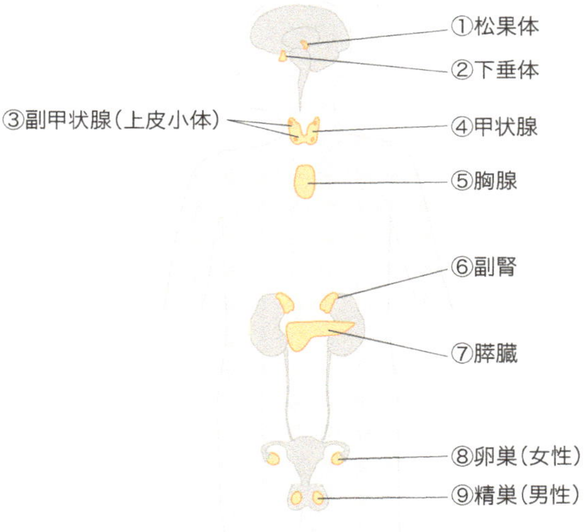

①松果体

②下垂体

③副甲状腺（上皮小体）

④甲状腺

⑤胸腺

⑥副腎

⑦膵臓

⑧卵巣（女性）

⑨精巣（男性）

Objectives of this Chapter　本章の目的

Anatomy and physiology	Understanding the functions and constituents of the endocrine system 内分泌系の機能と構成の理解
Disease	Learning pathology of hyperthyroidism 内分泌疾患・甲状腺機能亢進症の学習
Dialog	Discussing the suitable diet for hyperthyroidism 甲状腺機能亢進症の適切な食事について
Grammar review	Reviewing the tense of present, past, and future 現在形，過去形，未来形の復習

Anatomy and Physiology of the Endocrine System

内分泌系の解剖生理

Medical Terminology

adrenal gland	副腎(腎上体)
adrenalin	アドレナリン (副腎髄質で合成され交感神経などの興奮により分泌されるホルモン)
blood level	血中濃度
endocrine gland	内分泌腺
endocrine system	内分泌系
feedback loop	フィードバックループ
hypothalamus	視床下部
islet cell	(膵)島細胞
lipid	脂質
mammary gland	乳腺
nipple	乳首
nucleus (複数形nuclei)	細胞核(神経核)
oxytocin	オキシトシン (脳下垂体から分泌されるホルモン。授乳時に乳汁を出やすくするため分泌を促進する)
pancreas	膵臓
parathyroid gland	副甲状線(上皮小体)
pineal gland	松果体
pituitary	下垂体
placenta	胎盤
prolactin	プロラクチン (脳下垂体から分泌されるホルモン。妊娠, 出産に関わる)
receptor	受容体
testes (testisの複数形)	精巣(睾丸)
thyroid gland	甲状腺
thyroid stimulating hormone	甲状腺刺激ホルモン

Find answers to the following questions.　質問の答えを読み取ろう。

Q1. What is the endocrine system composed of?

Q2. What do the main endocrine glands include?

Q3. Does a small amount of hormone affect the body?

Q4. Where are the hormone receptors in the body?

Q5. What functions do the thyroid hormones formed in the thyroid glands have?

Q6. When and where is insulin formed?

Q7. What controls the secretion rate of pituitary hormone?

Q8. When is adrenalin produced?

The endocrine system is the collection of glands that regulate the activity of cells and organs. The endocrine system consists of the endocrine glands that produce and secrete hormones into the blood stream. The main endocrine glands include the hypothalamus, pituitary, thyroid gland, parathyroid gland, pineal gland, pancreas, adrenal glands, ovaries in women and testes in men. The hormones are the chemical substances affecting the works of the target parts of the body.

Even a small amount of hormones can cause a major reaction in the body. Hormones work as messengers, regulating and cooperating with the activities of each part of the body. Reaching the target organs, hormones combine with their receptors and transmit the information to the target organs to support special functions. The hormone receptors are located on the surface of the cells or in the nuclei.

Some hormones affect one or two organs, and others affect the whole body. For example, the thyroid stimulating hormones which are formed in the pituitary gland affect only the thyroid gland, while the thyroid hormones formed in the thyroid gland have important functions, such as affecting all cells in the body and their growth, controlling heart rate and influencing the consumption of calories needed for energy. Insulin secreted from the pancreatic islet affects the metabolism of glucose and lipid.

Many endocrine glands are controlled by the interplaying of hormonal signals of hormones between the hypothalamus and the pituitary in the brain. The hypothalamus secretes several kinds of hormones which control the pituitary. The pituitary is called the master gland which regulates other endocrine gland functions. The pituitary controls the rate at which it secretes hormones through a feedback loop. Through this mechanism, the blood levels of other endocrine hormones signal the pituitary to increase or decrease the rate of hormone secretion from the pituitary.

Many other factors can regulate endocrine functions. When babies suck on the nipple of its mother, the stimulation is transmitted to the pituitary, secreting prolactin and oxytocin which inform the breasts to produce and release milk. In the case of rising blood glucose level, insulin is produced by stimulating the islet cells in the pancreas. When the sympathetic nerves get excited, adrenalin is produced in the adrenal glands.

The disorders of endocrine system can result from hormone overproduction or underproduction.

Exercise Answer the illustrations ①~⑨ in English. p.49のイラストの①～⑨の各部位を英語で書きなさい。

・チアマゾール，プロピルチオウラシル：バセドウ病の甲状腺機能亢進症に効果がある薬。

・甲状腺クリーゼ：未治療または治療が不十分の甲状腺機能亢進症に関し，命に関わる疾患。患者の心拍，血圧，体温が危険な状態まで上昇し，迅速に治療されないと死にいたる。

Hyperthyroidism

内分泌疾患　甲状腺機能亢進症

Medical Terminology

arrhythmia	不整脈	irritability	怒りっぽいこと，短気
auto-antibody	自己抗体	methimazole	メチマゾール
bulge	突き出る	nodule	小結節，細胞小集合体
diplopia	複視，二重視	nucleus	細胞核
exophthalmos	眼球突出	perspiration	汗，発汗
eye socket	眼窩	propylthiouracil	プロピルチオウラシル
goiter	甲状腺腫	thyroid storm	甲状腺クリーゼ
Graves' disease	グレーブス病（バセドー病とも呼ばれる）	tremor	ふるえ
hyperthyroidism	甲状腺機能亢進症	undertreated	治療されていない
impairment	悪化，損傷		

Find answers to the following questions. 質問の答えを読み取ろう。

Q1. What is hyperthyroidism?

Q2. What is the main cause of hyperthyroidism?

Q3. What is goiter?

Q4. What are the symptoms of hyperthyroidism?

Q5. What are the special symptoms of Graves' disease?

Q6. What is the cause of exophthalmos?

Q7. What is thyroid storm crisis?

Hyperthyroidism is a disease caused by the excessive production of thyroid hormone by the thyroid gland, resulting in the increase of speed of the functions of the body. Though there may be other causes of hyperthyroidism, the main cause is Graves' disease. Graves' disease is an autoimmune disease caused by the auto-antibodies, which are produced by the person's immune system, binding to the receptors in the nucleus of thyroid cells, resulting in an overactive thyroid.

Those who have hyperthyroidism have an enlarged thyroid gland and this is called goiter. Common signs and symptoms of this disease are rapid heart rate, high blood pressure, arrhythmia, increase in perspiration, hand tremors, anxiety and irritability, increase of appetite and possible weight loss etc.

In the Graves' disease, in addition to the above symptoms exophthalmos and diplopia may appear. Exophthalmos is bulging of the eyes and is caused by inflammation inside the eye socket. Diplopia is visual impairment in which an object appears as two and is caused by inflammation in the eye.

The disease can be diagnosed through a physical examination, blood sample test, and a radioactive iodine uptake test to measure the amount taken up the thyroid. When the blood tests show a low thyroid stimulating hormone and a high thyroid gland hormone, the disease is confirmed.

Treatments depend on the severity of the disease. Anti-thyroid medications such as methimazole or propylthiouracil are often used, and the medications work by decreasing the production of thyroid hormone.

Thyroid storm is a life-threatening health condition of extreme hyperthyroidism which occurs suddenly. The disease occurs when hyperthyroidism goes untreated or is treated insufficiently. During thyroid storm a person's heart rate, blood pressure and body temperature rise to dangerous levels. The main cause of thyroid storm is undertreated severe hyperthyroidism accompanied by infection, inflammation, trauma from surgery and /or severe emotional stress.

Useful information ヨードと甲状腺の関係は？

ヨードには甲状腺ホルモンの産生，子供の成長ホルモン分泌を促進する働きがあり，体に必要な栄養素です。しかし，バセドウ病の人がヨードを取りすぎると，薬が効かなくなったりすることがあります。
ヨード（ヨウ素）を多く含む食品（海藻類が多い）…ひじき，昆布，わかめ，あおのり，天草など

Dialog about Basedow disease

バセドウ病についての対話

Basedow disease：バセドウ病またはバセドー病。

iodine：ヨード（ヨウ素）

A: Hey, nice to see you today. How have you been?

B: Not so good. I have been very tired recently, so I went to the clinic near my house and had some blood tests. I am so surprised at the results of blood tests. It showed I had Graves'disease.

A: Graves'disease? I don't know that disease.

B: I didn't, either. The doctor told me that the other name of the disease is Basedow disease, the excess work of endocrine gland causes the disease and more women have the disease than men.

A: Do you have any symptoms?

B: I have lost a lot of weight in spite of eating a lot and my hands tremble. I am not so worried because the disease doesn't seem to develop seriously in the body. I started some medication to decrease the hormone production in endocrine gland.

A: Can you still eat almost anything?

B: I can eat everything except food that includes a high amount of iodine. Seaweed contains a lot of iodine, so I'll have to try to eat western style diet with little iodine.

A: Japanese style diets often include much seaweed, so you should be safe with a western diet. Take care of yourself. I hope you get well soon.

B: Yes, thank you. I hope so, too.

Find answers to the following questions. 質問の答えを読み取ろう。

Q1. What is Graves' disease?

Q2. What are symptoms of Graves' disease?

Grammar Review 時制

時制とは動詞の語形変化によって時を表すものです。現在，過去，未来が基本時制。

時の流れ →
過去　現在　未来

現在時制（Present Tense）：現在の状態，習慣，不変の真理，近い未来を表す。

He lives in Canada now. He is a college student.

The sun is bigger than the earth. Two plus two is four.

My father comes back to Japan from the US tonight.

過去時制（Past Tense）：過去のあるときの動作，出来事，状態，過去の習慣を表す。

We visited our aunt and uncle yesterday.

A big earthquake occurred three years ago.

There used to be a park near my house when young.

未来時制（Future Tense）：未来の動作，出来事を表す。

I will go shopping tomorrow.

She will be busy cleaning the house for the party.

They are going to do a volunteer activity this Sunday.

注意すべき活用の動詞

- stand　stood　stood
- eat　ate　eaten
- take　took　taken
- get　got　gotten
- see　saw　seen
- fall　fell　fallen（倒れる）
- fell　felled　felled（倒す）
- find　found　found（見つける）
- found　founded　founded（設立する）

Exercise　Change a verb in (　) to a suitable form. (　)内の動詞を適切な形に変えなさい。

1. One of my friends always (clean) his room every day.
2. Tom (leave) Japan after staying for two weeks yesterday.
3. Mr. Smith (found) the Volunteer Club 20 years ago.
4. Ken (take) a bath every day.
5. John (try) to find the good medicine to cure chronic diseases now.

Chapter

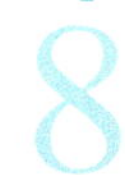

The Female Reproductive System
女性生殖器

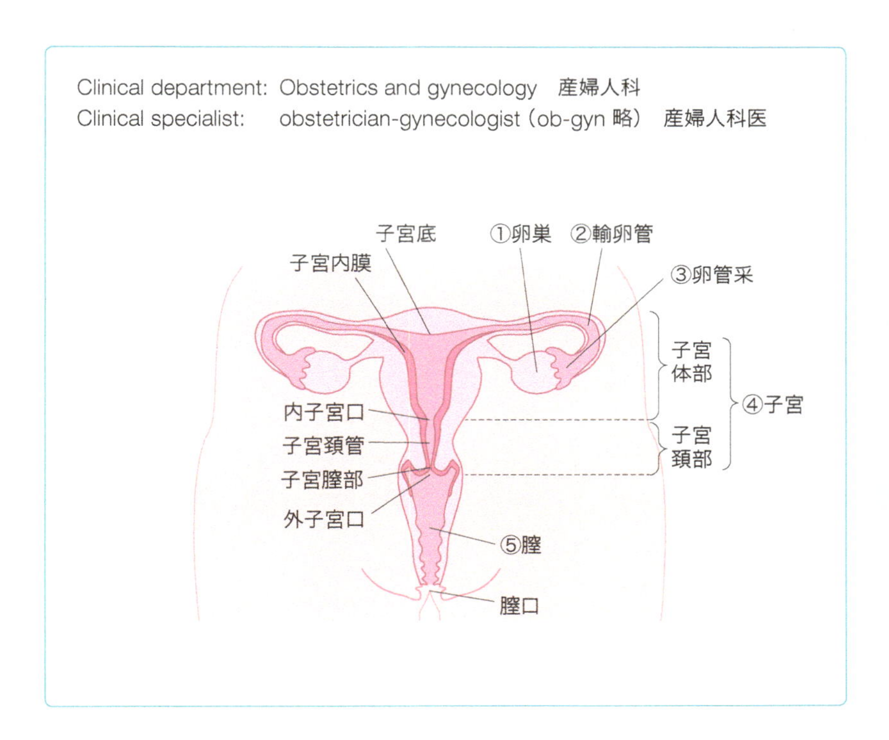

Objectives of this Chapter 本章の目的

Anatomy and physiology	Understanding the function and constituents of female reproductive system 女性生殖器の解剖生理の理解
Disease	Learning pathology of uterine fibroid 子宮筋腫の学習
Dialog	Discussing a breech baby 逆子について
Grammar review	Reviewing the present perfect and past perfect 現在完了・過去完了の復習

The Female Reproductive System

女性生殖器

Medical Terminology

cilia	線毛
clitoris	陰核(クリトリス)
embryo	胎芽(受精8週未満の生体)
endometrium	子宮内膜
fallopian tube	卵管
fertilized egg	受精卵
fetus	胎児
fimbriae	卵管采
follicle stimulating hormones	卵胞刺激ホルモン
genital tract	生殖器, 外性器
labia majora	大陰唇
labia minora	小陰唇
lining of the uterus	子宮内膜
menopause	更年期
menstrual cycle	月経周期
menstruation	月経
mons pubis	恥丘
ovaries (単数ovary)	卵巣
ovulation	排卵
ovum (複数形はova)	卵子
pituitary glands	下垂体
rectum	直腸
sperm	精子
uterine cervix	子宮頸管
uterine corpus	子宮体部
uterus	子宮
urine tube	卵管
vagina	膣
vulva	外陰部

Find answers to the following questions. 質問の答えを読み取ろう。

Q1. What do the external sex organs include?

Q2. What do the internal sex organs include?

Q3. What shape is the uterus?

Q4. Where does a fertilized egg grow?

Q5. Where does the male sperm meet the ova?

Q6. How does fimbria work for ova?

Q7. What kind of organ is the ovary?

Q8. How many ova do female newborns have?

Q9. What controls the menstrual cycle?

Q10. When does the menstrual cycle start and finish in one's life time?

The female reproductive system consists of the internal and external sex organs. The external organs include mons pubis, labia majora, labia minora and clitoris, which are called the vulva, located just outside the opening of the vagina. The breasts and mammary glands are included as part of the female reproductive system.

The internal reproductive organs are part of the genital tract, and are composed of the uterus, ovaries, fallopian tubes and vagina.

The vagina is the place where male sperms are released, and it serves as the birth canal during childbirth. It is connected to the uterine cervix.

The uterus is a pear-shaped muscular organ located between the urinary bladder and the rectum. The uterus also known as the womb supports the development of the embryo to a fetus during pregnancy. The uterus produces uterine secretions which help to carry the released sperm to the fallopian tubes. The fallopian tubes connect the ovaries to the uterus. Fertilization occurs in the fallopian tubes where sperms meet the eggs known as ova.

The uterine corpus is a thick wall organ made of muscle that gets bigger and bigger as the fetus grows. At the birth time, the fetus is pushed out by the contraction of the muscle and outside of the body through the birth canal (the vagina) from uterine cervix.

It is in the fallopian tube where sperms meet ova and fertilization occurs. At its end, the tube grows wider, becoming palm-shaped fimbriae. The fimbriae leads ova excreted from the ovary to the entrance of the fallopian tube. The inside of the fallopian tube is covered with thousands of cilia and the movement of these cilia help ova travel to the uterus.

The two ovaries are the organs where ova are produced and excreted. Ovulation is the process in which a single egg cell is released from the left or right ovary every 28 days or so. A newborn baby girl has one million egg cells in the ovary but only about 400 egg cells are released through her lifetime. The menstrual cycle is controlled through hormones. Follicle stimulating hormones released from the pituitary glands not only promote ovulation but also secrete estrogen and progesterone by stimulating the ovary. Estrogen and progesterone stimulate the uterus and the breasts, signaling them to prepare for fertilization. If the egg fails to get fertilized by a sperm, it is discharged along with the endometrium from the uterus. Menstruation is the term given to the periodic shedding of the endometrium. The blood and fluid excreted from the body passes through the cervix and vagina.

The female menstrual cycle takes about 24-35 days, depending on the individual. Menstruation begins during puberty, when the ovaries begin to produce more estrogen and other hormones, and this continues through to menopause. When almost all of the egg cells have died or have been released, the body starts its menopausal phase. Once menopause occurs, menstruation ceases.

Exercise Answer the illustrations ①~⑤ in English. p.57のイラストの①~⑤を英語で答えなさい。

Explain the steps for pregnant in English. 妊娠の過程を英語で説明しなさい。

1. 卵巣から卵子が排卵
2. 排卵した卵子が卵管に吸い上げられる
3. 精子の移動
4. 精子待機
5. 精子と卵子が受精
6. 胚分割
7. 着床
8. 妊娠
9. 出産

Uterine fibroid

子宮筋腫

Medical Terminology

benign	良性の
caesarean section	帝王切開
degeneration	変形
distort	ゆがめる，ねじる
endometrium	子宮内膜
gastrointestinal	胃腸の
GnRH	ゴナドトロピン放出ホルモンの略
hysterectomy surgery	子宮摘出術
intramural fibroids	筋層膜筋腫
lesion	病変
myomectomy (surgery)	筋腫核出術
submucosal fibroids	粘膜下筋腫
subserosal fibroids	漿膜下筋腫
uterine artery embolization (UAE)	子宮動脈閉塞術
uterine fibroid	子宮筋腫

Find answers to the following questions. 質問の答えを読み取ろう。

Q1. What kinds of tumor is a uterine fibroid?

Q2. What classifies uterine fibroids?

Q3. What is the most common type of fibroid?

Q4. When does a uterine fibroid get larger?

Q5. What symptoms do women have when fibroids get big?

Q6. Why may a woman with fibroid have a caesarean section operation?

Q7. How do doctors diagnose the fibroids?

Q8. Does every patient with fibroids need treatments?

Q9. What medicine is used to relieve the symptoms?

Q10. What operation is chosen when a patient wants to keep the uterus?

uterine artery embolization (UAE：子宮動脈閉塞術)　子宮筋腫の子宮を傷つけずに行う治療法。筋腫が成長するために必要な栄養が送られている血管を詰まらせることにより，筋腫を壊死させる方法。栄養血管に血管閉塞剤を注入し血管を閉塞させる。

A uterine fibroid is a benign smooth muscle tumor of the uterus, which about 70% of all women have. The size can vary from very small to the size of a basketball. Uterine fibroids are classified into different types by their location: intramural fibroids, subserosal fibroids and submucosal fibroids, etc.

Intramural fibroids are the most common type and are located within the muscular wall of the uterus. Subserosal fibroids are less common and are located on the surface of the uterus. Submucosal fibroids are the least common and are located in the muscle beneath the endometrium of the uterus. Fibroids usually increase in size during pregnancy due to an increase in hormone production, but decrease in size after menopause due to the falling levels of estrogen.

Most fibroids are relatively small and have no symptoms but in the case of submucosal fibroids, symptoms such as heavy menstrual bleeding may appear. This bleeding may result in anemia, a condition related to low blood iron. When fibroids increase in size and cause degeneration, they can create the feeling of tightness in abdomen, causing lower abdominal pain and other problems. Pressure to the bladder leads to frequent urination and the pressure to the intestinal tract leads to constipation. Fibroids can also cause infertility. Moreover when a woman with fibroids becomes pregnant, premature or a still birth may result. A caesarean section may be performed when a natural birth gets difficult due to fibroids. During pregnancy, fibroids increase in size and decrease after birth due to the rising and falling levels of hormone production. Fibroids are usually diagnosed through MRI and ultrasonography imaging techniques.

Most fibroids are benign, meaning noncancerous. Therefore, not all women need treatment. Symptom-free fibroids need not to be treated. But those with serious symptoms are usually treated with myomectomy or hysterectomy surgery. For those wishing to keep the uterus in order to become pregnant, myomectomy is the best choice. Medication such as gonadotropin (GnRH), a hormone production controller, may be used to relieve symptoms of bleeding and to decrease the size of fibroids. Uterine artery embolization (UAE), a relatively new treatment, may be performed in some cases. Women who have entered menopause do not necessarily need treatment since fibroids decrease in size once estrogen levels in the body decrease.

Dialog about a breech presentation

逆子についての対話

Medical Terminology

a breech presentation, a breech baby	骨盤位，逆子(さかご)	antenatal clinic	妊産婦健診医療機関
acupuncture treatment	鍼灸治療	pregnancy check-ups	妊婦健診

Mother (M) and her daughter Susan (S) are talking.

M: Good morning, Susan. Did you visit an antenatal clinic for pregnancy check-ups?

S: Oh, yes, Mom. At the clinic, the doctor told me my baby was 5 months and a breech baby. I was very surprised to hear what the doctor said. So I must have another checkup in a week.

M: Don't worry, Susan. Your baby will move to a normal position.

S: I hope so. My friend's baby was a breech baby, but moved to a normal position and no more to a breech position.

M: That's good! Recently I have read an article that acupuncture treatment works well for a breech baby. Moreover WHO recognizes the acupuncture effects for some cases.

S: Really?

M: You should visit the acupuncture clinic which my friend runs. I will make an appointment for you today.

S: Thank you so much. I am very relieved to hear your advice. I will visit the clinic tomorrow.

Find answers to the following questions. 質問の答えを読み取ろう。

Q1. Why does Susan worry about her baby?

Q2. What treatment works for a breech baby?

Grammar Review
現在完了（present perfect）と過去完了（past perfect）

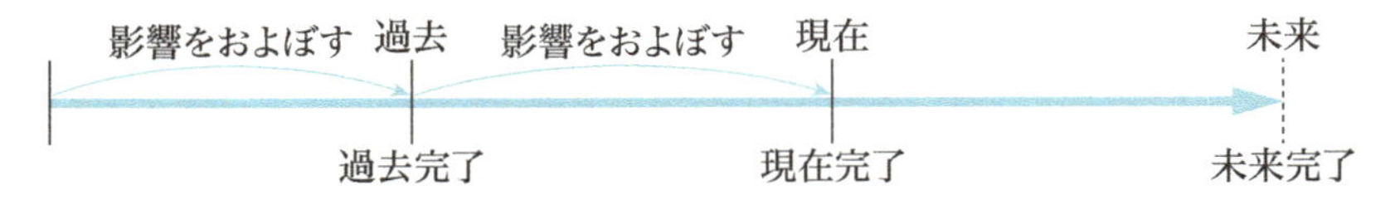

現在完了　過去に起こった動作，状態が現在結びついている状態。

have (has) ＋過去分詞

1）動作・出来事の完了：I have finished my work.

2）経験：Have you ever seen such a big gorilla?

I have never been to New York.

3）現代までの継続：

I have known her since I was a child.

She has cleaned the house since morning. (has been cleaning)

＊継続を強く表現するときは現在完了進行形にする。have＋ been ＋〜動詞 ing

過去完了　**had ＋過去分詞**

1）過去のある時までの動作・状態の完了・結果

The bus had already left when I arrived at the bus stop.

2）過去のある時までの状態の継続

My grandfather had been sick for a few days when he was carried to hospital.

3）過去のある時よりも前の動作・出来事

I lost my purse which my parents had given me for my birthday.

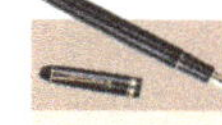

Useful information 鍼治療って？

鍼治療が痛みを緩和することはよく知られており，実際に頭痛，生理痛，癌慢性疼痛などの痛みに対しては鍼治療が応用されています。中国では数千年にわたる実践によって築かれた「中国医学」の理論に基づき，さまざまな疾患治療に鍼治療が使用されています。鍼治療応用疾患として1996年にWHOが41の疾患を発表しています（テニス肘，捻挫，高血圧，不整脈，下痢症，便秘症，胆石症など）。逆子にも効果があるとされています。

Chapter 9 The Skeletal System

骨格系

Clinical department: Orthopedics　整形外科
Clinical specialist: Orthopedic surgeon or Orthopedist　整形外科医
surgeon　外科医

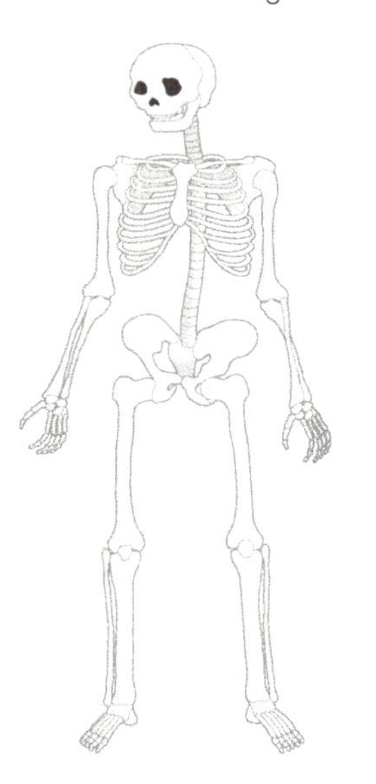

骨：上肢

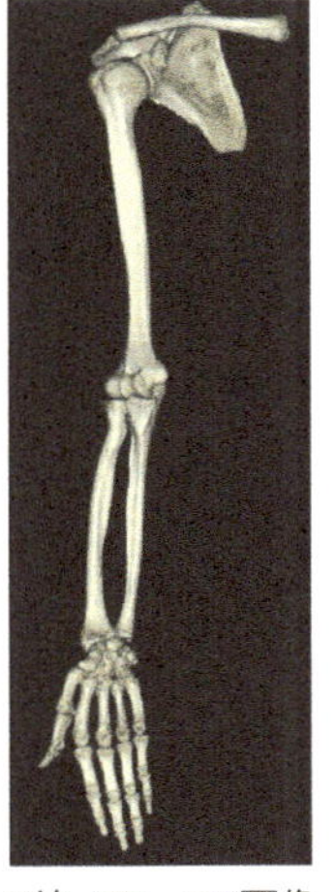

X線-CT　3D画像

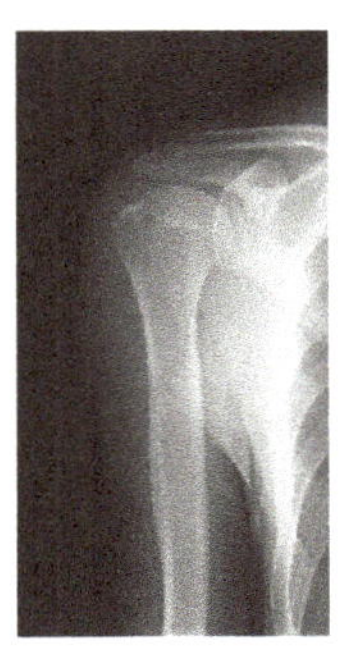

単純X線写真

Objectives of this Chapter　本章の目的

Anatomy and physiology	Understanding functions of the skeletal system 骨格系の機能理解
Disease	Learning about spinal disc herniation 椎間板ヘルニアの学習
Dialog	Discussing the treatments of spinal disc herniation 椎間板ヘルニアの治療について
Grammar review	Reviewing auxiliary verbs 助動詞の復習

The Skeletal System

骨格系

Medical Terminology

articular capsule	関節包
biaxial joint	二軸性関節
bone morphogeny	骨形成
capsular ligament	関節包靭帯
carpal bone	手根骨
cartilage plate	軟骨板
compact bone	緻密骨
compound joint	複合関節
condyloid joint (ellipsoid joint)	楕円関節
endochondral ossification	内軟骨性骨化
extracapsular ligament	関節包外靭帯
facial cranium	顔面頭蓋（がんめんとうがい）
femur	大腿骨
fixed joint	不動関節
hinge joint	蝶番関節
humerus (複数形はhumeri)	上腕骨
ilium	腸骨
intramembranous ossification	膜性骨化
irregular bone	不規則骨
joint cavity	関節腔
ligament	靭帯
long columnar	長円柱形
marrow	骨髄
maxillary bone (maxilla)	上顎骨
movable joint	可動関節
multiaxial joint	多軸性関節
patellae (単数形はpatella)	膝蓋骨
patellar ligament	膝蓋靭帯
pivot	軸
plane joint	平面関節
pneumatized bone	含気骨
saddle joint	鞍関節
scapula	肩甲骨
sesamoid bone	種子骨
simple joint	単関節
skull	頭蓋骨
sphenoid	蝶形骨
spherical joint (ball and socket joint)	球関節
sternoclavicular joint	胸鎖関節
synovial fluid	滑液
synovial membrane	滑膜
tarsal bone	足根骨
tendon	腱
trochoid joint	車軸関節
uniaxial joint	一軸性関節
vertebra (複数形は vertebrae)	椎体

Find answers to the following questions. 質問の答えを読み取ろう。

Q1. What are the bones made of?

Q2. What functions do the bones have?

Q3. How many bones are in the body?

Q4. Name the five kinds of bones.

Q5. What is the biggest bone in the sesamoid bone?

Q6. When does the growth of bones stop in men?

Q7. How are joints classified?

Q8. What functions do ligaments have?

Bones are hard solid living organs made of fibers and minerals. Bones have some important functions: helping to support the body structure, protecting certain parts of body, making blood in the marrow and storing minerals.

The body has 206 bones and these are listed as follows:

1. Long bones: The shapes of these bones are a long columnar with both ends getting bigger. (ex. humerus, femur)
2. Short bones: They are short and mostly composed of spongy bones. (ex. carpal bone, tarsal bone)
3. Flat bones: The shape of the bones is flat with thin layer of spongy bone enclosed within the two thin layers of compact bones. (ex. skull, ilium)
4. Irregular bones: The shape of the bones is irregular. (ex. scapula, vertebra)
5. Pneumatized bones: These bones have a cavity of air inside. (ex. maxilla, sphenoid)

Small round bones which grow in a tendon or ligament are called sesamoid bones. The biggest sesamoid bones are the patellae which exist in patellar ligaments.

The growth of the bones is aided by intramembranous ossification and endochondral ossification. The former is bone morphogeny by bone membrane as in the skull and ilium. The latter is bone morphogeny of growth cartilage plate as in the femur and humerus. These bones commonly continue to grow until the age of seventeen or eighteen in males and age of fifteen or sixteen in females.

The structural substance connected between two or more bones is called joint and these joints link the skeletal system into a functional whole. Joints are classified by bone numbers and their movements. Joints composed of two bones are called simple joints and those constructed of three or more bones are called compound joints.

Joints are classified into three by their movements: uniaxial joints moving on a special pivot, biaxial joints moving on two pivots, and multiaxial joints moving on three or more pivots and in all directions.

Moreover joints are classified into movable joints and fixed joints.

Most joints of the four limbs (upper and lower limbs) are the movable joints, which are covered with synovial membrane inside and keep synovial fluid in the cavity of the joints, therefore they are called synovial joints.

Fixed joints do not have synovial membrane, joint cavity nor synovial fluid. Connective tissues exist between the bones, which constitute the fixed joints. The stemoclavicular joint is this type.

Joints are also classified by the shape: spherical joint (ball and socket joint), saddle joint, trochoid joint (pivot joint), condyloid joint (ellipsoid joint), hinge joint and plane joint (flat joint).

Ligaments are important tissues for composing joints which connect bones. Their functions are both fixing joints and controlling the range of the joints. Capsular ligaments increase the strength of joints with articular capsule and extracapsular ligaments work for stabilizing the joints with protecting the separation of bones.

骨の分類 the classification of the bones

長骨	the long bones	humerus
短骨	the short bones	carpal bones, tarsal bones
扁平骨	the flat bones	skull
不規則骨	the irregular bones	vertebra
含気骨	the pneumatized bones	maxilla

Spinal disc herniation

椎間板ヘルニア

Medical Terminology

achilles tendon reflex	アキレス腱反射	motor paralysis	運動麻痺
anti-inflammatory analgestic	消炎鎮痛剤	muscle weakness	筋力低下
bladder rectal disorder	膀胱直腸障害	nucleus palposus	髄核
block therapy	ブロック療法	numbness	しびれ
cartilaginous	軟骨性	painful sensation	疼痛
corset	コルセット	preservation therapy	保存療法
disorder of sensation	知覚障害	radiating pain	放散痛
endoscopic surgery	内視鏡手術	rear discectomy	後方椎間板切除術
epidual block	硬膜外ブロック	sensational desensitization	知覚鈍麻
fibrous	繊維性	spinal cord	脊髄
fibrous rings	繊維輪	spinal disc herniation	椎間板ヘルニア
hyperthermia therapy	温熱療法	spinal discs	椎間板
intermittent traction therapy	間欠牽引療法	the cervical disc herniation	頚椎椎間板ヘルニア
Lasegues's sign (straight leg raising test)	ラセーグ徴候，坐骨グラフィー	the tests of kneecap reflex	膝蓋腱反射テスト
love method	ラブ法	vertebral body	椎体
malformation	奇形	vertebral body of spine	脊椎の椎体

Find answers to the following questions. 質問の答えを読み取ろう。

Q1. What condition is spinal disc herniation?

Q2. What are the symptoms of the cervical disc herniation?

Spinal discs are the strong tissues existing between the vertebrae of the spine and vertebral body and are composed of fibrous rings and cartilaginous nucleus palposus (the gel-like substance that allows slight movement of the vertebrae). Spinal disc herniation, also known as a slipped disc, is a condition in which a rupture of a fibrous ring of spinal disc causes the nucleus palposus to swell up and bulge out the spinal canal. This causes painful sensations and some symptoms related with nerves. The cervical disc herniation is the condition where both the spinal cords and nerve roots are compressed and causes symptoms such as neck pain, muscle weakness of lower limbs, bladder rectal disorder, disorder of sensation in the upper limbs and radiating pain in the upper limbs as nerve root symptoms. Lumbar disc herniation doesn't cause any spinal disc symptoms but causes numbness, muscle weakness, radiating pain in the lower limbs or bladder rectal disorder.

This disease is diagnosed by patient's symptoms and also through tests of kneecap reflex, achilles tendon reflex, sensational desensitization in lower limbs and Lasegues's sign. A simple X-ray examination, CT, MRI, and/or Myelography are used for image examinations diagnosis. MRI is notably the best for diagnosing a herniated disc and its malformation as it has the clearest image and has the least negative effect on the body.

The treatment for minor herniated discs is preservation therapy meaning physical therapy or exercise but severe herniated discs require surgery. Patients often recover within three months by getting physical therapy or exercise therapy. In the case of acute(r) phase, medical therapy using anti-inflammatory anesthetic (analgestic) or block therapy of an epidural (epidural block) is offered to inpatients. After patients' symptoms improve, hyperthermia therapy, intermittent index therapy or wearing of soft corset is recommended to outpatients.

Surgery is rarely required, however it is recommended to those who develop motor paralysis or show no improvement after physical therapy or exercise within 3 months. The most common style of surgery is rear discectomy, so -called love method. Nowadays endoscopic surgery is introduced, which helps patients recover sooner with a less burden on the body.

Dialog at the acupuncture clinic

鍼灸クリニックでの対話

Acupuncturist (A): Hello. What brought you here today?

Ken (K): I have had terrible pain for a week. The symptoms are getting worse and worse recently, so I have not been able to walk nor stand for a long time.

A: Oh, that is no good. Please relax and I will check your pulse and your tongue condition.

K: Can you understand my body condition just by checking my tongue and pulse?

A: Yes, your tongue and your pulse show your body condition clearly.
The diagnosis method by examining your tongue and pulse is based on the theory of Traditional Chinese Medicine (TCM) which was established 3000 years ago. We acupuncturists treat patients with the knowledge of both western and eastern medicine. I am sure acupuncture treatment works for pain the best.
But I wonder if your lower back pain is caused by a spinal disc herniation or some other causes. You had better have your spinal disc examined by an x-ray. I can treat you after considering the result of your x-ray.

K: Thank you so much for your advice. I will have an x-ray taken at the hospital tomorrow and then visit you again with the result.

A: Take care.

Find answers to the following questions. 質問の答えを読み取ろう。

Q1. Why did Ken visit the Acupuncture clinic?

Q2. How did an acupuncturist diagnose the patient?

Q3. Will Ken have an x-ray taken?

Grammar Review 助動詞（auxiliary verb）

助動詞は動詞の一種で，動詞に結びついて可能，義務，時制，などを表す。

助動詞＋動詞の原形　可能，推量，許可，義務，未来，意志などを表す（can, may, must, should, would, need, etc.）。

can: I can (am able to) finish my report.

may: You may play here.

must: You must (have to) be quiet at the hospital.

should: You should be kind to the patients.

need: We need to get as much medical knowledge as we can.

助動詞を含む慣用表現

cannot ～ too ...：どんなに～してもしすぎることはない

You cannot praise your students too much.

may well ～：～するのはもっともだ，たぶん～するだろう

You may well be careful in crossing the busy road.

would rather ～ than ...：…するより～するほうがよい

I would rather stay at home than go out on a (the) rainy day.

would (should) like to ～：～したいものだ

I would like to eat Japanese cuisine.

Exercise　Fill in the blanks with suitable English word. 日本文に合うように空欄に適する語を入れなさい。

1. He (　　　) well do such things.（～するのは当然です）
2. You (　　　) (　　　) too careful in choosing your friends.
   （～しすぎることはない）
3. I (　　　) (　　　) to go abroad for getting much knowledge.（～したい）
4. You (　　　) study in order to be a good medical specialist.（～すべき）
5. She (　　　) be late for the class because of the accident.（～かもしれない）

Chapter

10 The Skeletal Muscles and the Tendons

骨格筋と腱

Clinical department: Orthopedic surgery 整形外科
Clinical specialist: Orthopedic surgeon 整形外科医

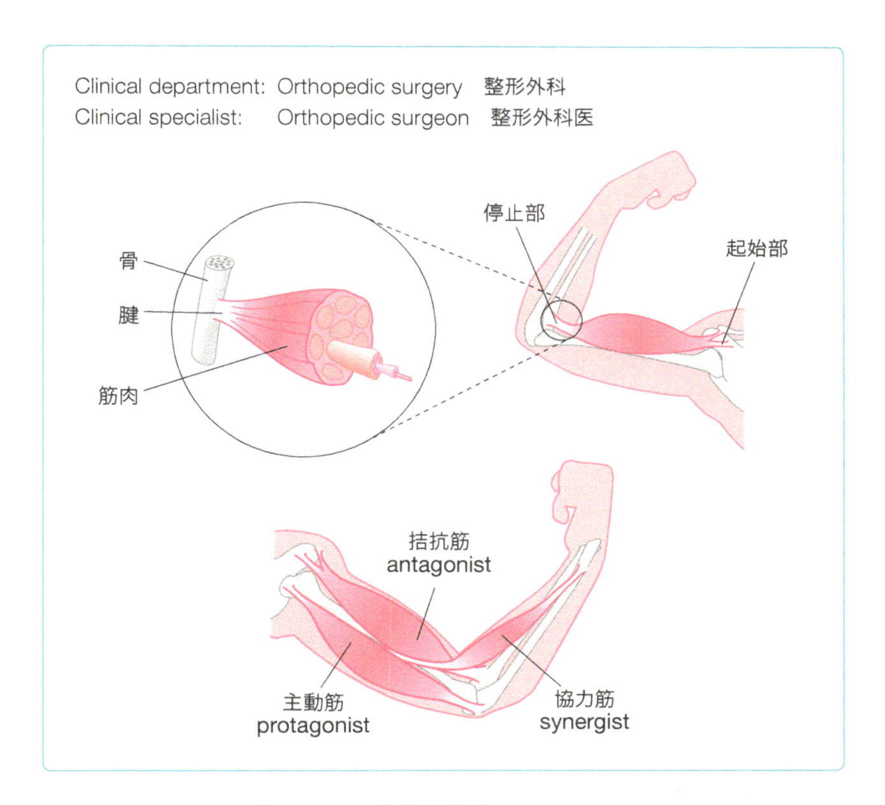

Objectives of this Chapter 本章の目的

Anatomy and physiology	Understanding the skeletal muscles and the tendons 筋肉や腱の理解
Disease	Learning pathology of Duchenne muscular dystrophy デュシェンヌ型筋ジストロフィー症の学習
Dialog	Discussing muscle types 筋肉の種類についての対話
Grammar review	Reviewing the passive voice form 受動態について復習する

Anatomy and Physiology of the Skeletal Muscles and the Tendons

骨格筋と腱の解剖生理

Medical Terminology

actin filament	アクチンフィラメント
antagonist	拮抗筋
antigravity muscle	抗重力筋
collagen	コラーゲン
contract	収縮する
distal	遠位(の)
joint	関節
lateral	横の
muscle spindle	筋紡錘
myofibril	筋原線維
myofilament	筋細糸(筋フィラメント)
myoglobin	ミオグロビン
origin	起始
overextend	過伸展する
protagonist	主動筋
proximal	近位(の)
red muscle	赤筋
skeletal muscle	骨格筋
spinal column	脊柱
stop	停止
striated muscle	横紋筋
synergist	協力筋
tendon	腱
tendon spindle (Golgi tendon organ)	腱紡錘(ゴルジ腱器官)
voluntary muscle	随意筋
white muscle	白筋

Find answers to the following questions. 質問の答えを読み取ろう。

Q1. What are the skeletal muscles attached to?

Q2. What is the function of skeletal muscle?

Q3. Which moves more, the origin or the stop of the skeletal muscle?

Q4. What regulates the speed or strength of the motion against the protagonist?

Q5. Which muscle helps in the sitting or standing position against gravity?

Q6. What color is the muscle that contains a lot of myoglobin?

Q7. What do bundles of myofilaments construct?

Q8. What is shown as lateral stripes of a skeletal muscle?

Q9.What senses muscle tension and prevents muscle overextension?

Skeletal muscles are voluntary muscles which help move the joints and the spinal column, most of which are attached to the bones by tendons and some to skin or other skeletal muscles. The skeletal muscles are also used to maintain posture against the force of gravity, to produce and store energy, to protect internal organs and so on.

The proximal region where a skeletal muscle attaches to the bone is called the origin and moves the least while the distal region of a muscle attached to the next bone is called the stop which moves the most in motion. The protagonist is the muscle that contracts primarily to produce the physical movement with the synergist which voluntarily cooperates with the prime mover. The antagonist works against the protagonist to regulate the speed or strength of the motion. The muscle which helps keep the sitting or standing position against the pressure of gravity is called the antigravity muscle.

Skeletal muscle is classified into red muscle and white muscle. Red muscle contains a high quantity of capillaries with more oxygen, myoglobin and mitochondria. Red muscle can continue activity and contract for longer periods of time whereas white muscle is used for speed and force. One skeletal muscle cell includes thousands of myofibrils which are 1-2 μm in diameter. Myofibrils are systematically constructed bundles of myofilaments which are arranged alternately between the thin actin filaments and the thick ones forming lateral stripes called striated muscles.

The tendon, which is a bundle of collagen fibers and located between the skeletal muscle and the bone, receives and transmits signals to contract the muscle to begin or stop a physical motion. The tendon spindle (the Golgi tendon organ) in a tendon as well as the muscle spindle in a muscle senses the muscle tension preventing a muscle from overextending.

Exercise Fill in the blanks. 空所に適語を入れなさい。

1. (   ) muscle … activities with speed and force
2. (   ) muscle … longer-term continuous activity

Duchenne Muscular Dystrophy

デュシェンヌ型筋ジストロフィー症

Medical Terminology

Achilles tendon	アキレス腱
ADL (activities of daily living)	日常生活動作
articular	関節の
Becker type	ベッカー型
buttock	臀部
congenital	先天性の
contracture	拘縮
Duchenne type	デュシェンヌ型
electromyography	筋電図検査
facioscapulohumeral	顔面肩甲上腕型
fatty degeneration	脂肪変性
gastrostomy	胃瘻造設
Gowers sign	ガワーズ兆候 (登攀性起立)
hereditary disease	遺伝性疾患
intubation feeding	経管栄養
limb-girdle type	肢体型
lumbar flexure	腰椎前弯
motor disturbance	運動障害
muscle biopsy	筋生検
muscular atrophy	筋萎縮
muscular dystrophy	筋ジストロフィー
progressive	進行性の
proximal limbs	四肢近位
pseudohypertrophy	仮性肥大
respiratory failure	呼吸不全
sex chromosome	性染色体
stem cell transplantation	幹細胞移植療法
thigh	大腿
toe walking (equine gait)	尖足歩行
tracheostomy	気管切開
triceps surae	下腿三頭筋
ventilator	人工呼吸器
waddling gait	動揺性歩行 (アヒル歩行)

Find answers to the following questions. 質問の答えを読み取ろう。

Q1. What type of muscular dystrophy occurs most often in Japan?

Q2. In what muscle is weakness specifically seen in muscular dystrophy?

Q3. When do you see symptoms of Gowers?

Q4. What do weakened muscles of the pharynx and larynx cause?

Q5. What confirms the diagnosis of muscular dystrophy?

Q6. What is the main therapy for a patient with muscular dystrophy?

Q7. How are ADL and QOL of a muscular dystrophy patient improved?

Muscular dystrophy is mainly a hereditary disease characterized by progressive muscular atrophy and muscle weakness. This disease is classified into several types such as Duchenne, which is severe and appears most often in Japan, benign Becker, congenital, limb-girdle, and facioscapulohumeral (FSHD) muscular dystrophy.

Duchenne type muscular dystrophy, occuring 1 in 3,500 boys, is typically inherited through abnormal sex chromosomes which interfere with protein production needed to form healthy muscle tissue. Parents often notice a child's disorder nearer to the age of three or four when their manner of walking is strange or different, they fall down easily or cannot run.

Muscle weakness of muscular dystrophy is especially noticeable in muscles of the proximal limbs such as in the thighs, upper arms and trunk. When patients try to stand up, they follow the motions which are called Gowers sign, namely, first they lie on their stomach, next they push up the buttocks with their hands on the floor, and then they raise their upper body supported by their hands climbing up the anterior parts of their thighs. They show lumbar flexure and waddling gait when they walk, and have psuedohypertrophy in the triceps surae caused by fatty degeneration. Moreover, the complete contracture of the triceps surae, the shortened Achilles tendon and others, cause toe walking (equine gait).

Patients' gradually weakened muscles make it difficult to walk for most patients by the time they are 8 or 9 years of age. They become confined to a wheelchair from about the age of 10 and many need permanent full-time assistance in order to live from their adolescence. In more severe progressive cases, weakened muscles of the pharynx and larynx cause eating and swallowing disorders, while the weakened respiratory muscles cause breathing disorders.

Duchenne type muscular dystrophy disease can be diagnosed by a medical history and physical examination, and blood biochemical examinations in many cases. If dystrophin gene deficiency is found through a genetic test, then it confirms a definite diagnosis.

Unfortunately, there is no cure for any form of dystrophy although treatments including stem cell transplantation and pharmacotherapy may slow its progression. Therefore, physical therapy is mainly offered to help maintain muscular strength and to ease articular contracture so as to improve the ability to sit upright, stand or even walk. Furthermore, it is important to improve activities of daily living (ADL) and quality of life (QOL) by arranging mobility aides equipment at home or school. As the disease progresses further, intubation feeding or a gastrostomy and a tracheostomy or a ventilator may be needed.

Patients with Duchenne type muscular dystrophy have a life expectancy of 10 to 20 years. Patients have often died of heart or respiratory failure around 20 years of age, however medical technology is said to have extended the life prognosis of the disease by approximately 10 years.

Exercise Fill with the explanation a) ~ d) for each illustration and put the number 1 ~ 4 to show the process of Gowers sign. 図の説明文をa〜dから選んで記号で答え，登攀性起立の順序に番号1〜4をつけなさい。

Explanation for the illustration			
number (　)	number (　)	number (　)	number (　)

a) Pushing up the buttocks with their hands on the floor

b) Climbing up the anterior parts of their thighs

c) Lying on their stomach

d) Raising their upper body supported by their hands

Dialog about Muscle Types

筋肉の種類についての対話

Match the terms and the illustrations. 図と意味を結びなさい。

骨格筋 （随意筋，横紋あり）	・	・ cardiac muscle ・	・
心筋 （不随意筋，横紋あり）	・	・ smooth muscle ・	・
平滑筋 （不随意筋，横紋なし）	・	・ skeletal muscle ・	・

Teacher (T): Can you tell me what the three kinds of muscles are?

Student (S): Yes. They are the skeletal, smooth and cardiac muscles.

T: That's right. What do you know about the skeletal muscle?

S: We can move our bodies thanks to the skeletal muscles. They are voluntary muscles, namely, we can make them move with our intention.

T: Yes, that's right. Do you remember what other functions skeletal muscles have?

S: Well, the other main functions are to keep our physical posture and to make or store energy.

T: Very good. Then what muscle is similar to the skeletal muscle?

S: The cardiac muscle is, because both of them are striated.

T: Great! How about smooth muscle and cardiac muscle?

S: They are both involuntary and we can't control their movement with our intension.

Exercise Indicate if these are true (T) or false (F). 対話文の内容に合っている（T）か，合っていない（F）か答えなさい。

1. One function of smooth muscle is to keep posture.
2. The cardiac muscle and smooth muscle are striated.
3. Involuntary muscles are the skeletal muscle and smooth muscle.

Grammar Review 受動態（受け身：passive voice）

通常の「～する，～である」という意味を表す「能動態」に対し，「～される」という受け身の意味を表すために，述語動詞の部分を「be動詞＋動詞の過去分詞形」にします。時制（現在・過去・未来など）はbe動詞の部分で区別します。

A dietitian prepares a therapeutic diet.
栄養士が治療食を準備する。

A therapeutic diet is prepared by a dietitian.
治療食が栄養士によって準備される。

A medical technologist examined the blood.
臨床検査技師が血液を検査した。

The blood was examined by a medical technologist.
血液は臨床検査技師によって検査された。

The physical therapist will stretch the patient's tendon.
理学療法士はその患者の腱を伸ばすだろう。

The patient's tendon will be stretched by the physical therapist.
その患者の腱は理学療法士によって伸ばされるだろう。

The radiological technologist is taking an X-ray.
その診療放射線技師がレントゲン写真を撮っているところだ。

An X-ray is being taken by the radiological technologist.
レントゲン写真がその診療放射線技師によって撮られているところだ。

Exercise Change the English into the passive voice from the following sentences and write their meaning in Japanese. 次の文を受動態にし，意味を答えなさい。

1. The doctor explains the method of treatment.
2. The pharmacist has created a new medicine.
3. An acupuncturist will treat his back pain.
4. An occupational therapist retrained the patient who had a walking problem.
5. A nurse is checking the patient's condition.

Chapter 11

The Central Nervous System

中枢神経系

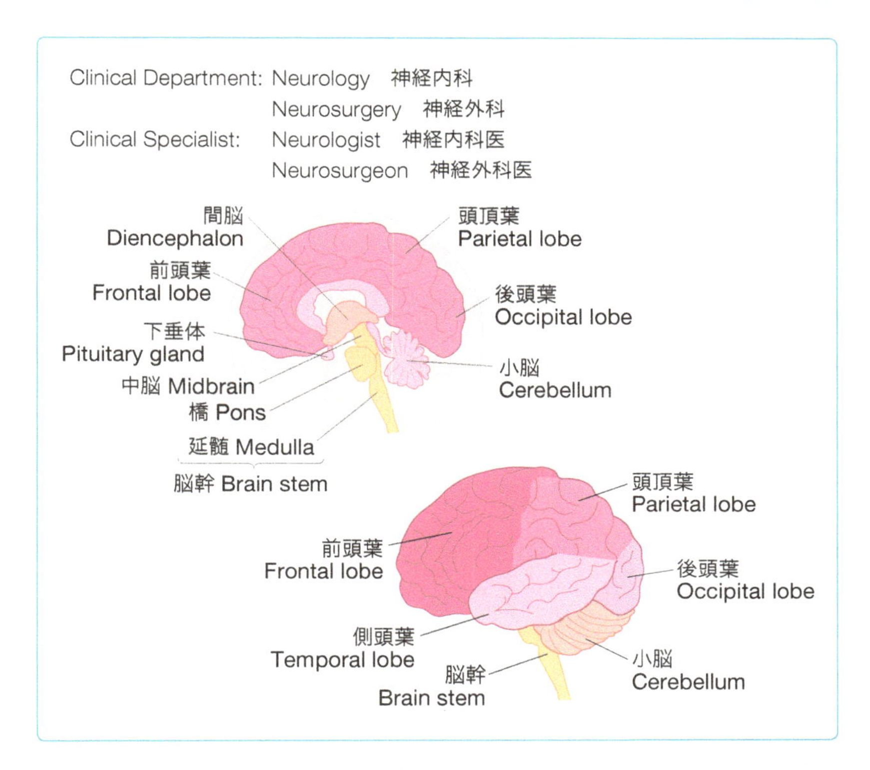

Objectives of this Chapter 本章の目的

Anatomy and physiology	Understanding the functions and the constituents of the central nervous system 中枢神経系の機能と構造を理解する
Disease	Learning the pathology of the central nervous system 中枢神経系の病理について学ぶ
Dialog	Talking about an operation and a central nervous disorder 中枢神経系の手術に関する対話
Grammar review	Reviewing the positive, comparative and superlative degree 原級, 比較級, 最上級について復習する

Anatomy and Physiology of the Nervous System

神経系の解剖生理

Medical Terminology

association fiber	連合線維	marrow	髄質
autonomic nervous system	自律神経系	medulla	延髄
basal ganglia	大脳基底核	midbrain	中脳
brain stem	脳幹	motor fiber	運動線維
caudate nucleus	尾状核	muscle tonus	筋トーヌス
central nervous system	中枢神経系	occipital lobe	後頭葉
cerebellum	小脳	pallidum	淡蒼球
cerebral hemisphere	大脳半球	parietal lobe	頭頂葉
cerebral sulcus	脳溝	peripheral nervous system	末梢神経系
cerebrum	大脳	pons	橋
commissural fibers	交連線維	projection fiber	投射線維
corpus callosum	脳梁	putamen	被殻
cortex	皮質	sensory fiber	感覚線維
diencephalon	間脳	spinal cord	脊髄
epithalamus	視床上部	striatum	線条体
fornix	脳弓	subthalamus	腹側視床
frontal lobe	前頭葉	telencephalon	終脳
gray matter	灰白質	temporal lobe	側頭葉
hypothalamus	視床下部	thalamus	視床
lenticular nucleus	レンズ核	voluntary movement	随意運動
longitudinal cerebral fissure	大脳縦裂	white matter board	白質板

Find answers to the following questions. 質問の答えを読み取ろう。

Q1. What does the nervous system comprise?

Q2. What does the central nervous system include?

Q3. What are the three nerve fibers and what do they do?

Q4. What makes the cerebral white matter's color white?

Q5. What functions does the cerebral gray matter have?

Q6. What does the basel ganglia include?

The nervous system comprises the central nervous system and peripheral nervous system. The central nervous system includes the brain and spinal cord. (We will explain the peripheral nervous system in chapter 12.) The brain is separated into the cerebellum and cerebrum, and the cerebrum has the telencephalon, diencephalon, and brain stem.

In this chapter, we will focus on the function of the telencephalon.

1. Cerebrum

1) telencephalon (cerebral hemisphere)

The telencephalon is devided into right and left cerebral hemispheres by the longitudinal cerebral fissure. The corpus callosum is located along the bottom of the longitudinal cerebral fissure. It is the white matter board which communicates between right and left cerebral hemispheres. There is the fornix under the corpus callosum. It is divided into the gray matter (cortex) and white matter (marrow). The gray matter is on the outside surface, and the white matter inside. The gray matter includes many nerve cell bodies, so its color is gray. Whereas the white matter includes many fibers, which contain much fat, therefore its color is white. In the white matter, there is gray matter which is a bunch of nerve cell bodies, and this is called the basal ganglia.

a) Cerebral gray matter

This is the area densely populated with nerve cell bodies, and in charge of the higher brain functions, such as perception, voluntary movement, thought, deduction, memory, etc. This is separated into the frontal lobe, parietal lobe, temporal lobe and occipital lobe by the cerebral sulci. The frontal lobe is in charge of thought, judgement, motion, and language processing. The parietal lobe is in charge of body sensation, language understanding, and the sense of taste. The temporal lobe is in charge of hearing, and language understanding.

The occipital lobe controls vision.

b) Cerebral white matter

The white matter includes the myelinated fiber of the neurons and the neuroglial cells (Especially the oligodendrocytes). The white matter is surrounded by the cortex, cerebral ventricle, and striatum (the caudate nucleus and the putamen). The neurons communicate with each other via nerve fibers. There are three kind of nerve fibers: the projection fiber which communicates between the relatively distant neurons, the association fiber which communicates within the same hemisphere, and the commissural fiber which communicates between right and left cerebral hemispheres.

c) Basal ganglia

The basal ganglia include the caudate nucleus, putamen, and pallidum. The caudate nucleus and the putamen are jointly called the striatum, and the putamen and the pallidum jointly called the lenticular nucleus, which are in charge of motion adjustment, cognition, emotion, motivation and learning. Its main function is motion initiation and motion acceleration, as well as the suppression of motion execution.

2) Diencephalon

The diencephalon is positioned between the brain stem and the telencephalon. It includes the thalamus, epithalamus, subthalamus and hypothalamus.

3) Brain stem

The brain stem is composed of the midbrain, pons and medulla.

2. Cerebellum

The cerebellum controls keeping right posture and balance, muscle tonus and voluntary motion.

3. Spinal cord

The spinal cord includes spinal nerves and some kinds of sensory and the motor fibers.

Brain hemorrhage

脳出血

Medical Terminology

antihypertensive therapy	降圧治療	hematoma	血腫
aphasia	失語症	internal capsule	内包
apraxia	失行	intracranial hypertension	頭蓋内圧亢進
arteriosclerosis	動脈硬化	myosis	縮瞳
brain edema	脳浮腫	oligodendrocyte	乏突起神経膠細胞
brain herniation	脳ヘルニア	osmotic diuretic	浸透圧性利尿薬
cerebral arteriovenous malformation	脳動静脈奇形	platelet disorder	血小板異常
coagulation disorder	凝固機能異常	quadriplegia	四肢麻痺
emergency craniotomy	緊急開頭術	subarachnoidal hemorrhage	くも膜下出血

Find answers to the following questions. 質問の答えを読み取ろう。

Q1. What is a brain hemorrhage?

Q2. What is the main cause of a brain hemorrhage?

Q3. What kinds of complications does brain hemorrhage have?

Q4. What are the symptoms of a brain hemorrhage?

Q5. What are the treatment options for a patient who has suffered a brain hemorrhage?

Q6. How is a brain hemorrhage diagnosed?

Q7. What is a hematoma?

A brain hemorrhage is bleeding into the brain tissue caused by bursting of blood vessels in the brain. This blood clot can develop into hematoma which makes brain dysfunction by damaging the local brain cells and by pressuring surrounding tissue.

The most likely cause of hemorrhage is vascular disruption due to high blood pressure or arteriosclerosis. Under the cause, there are some factors, which are as follows: the natural environment such as hot or cold outside temperature, social and psychological environment like heavy workloads and interpersonal stress, and personal habits such as smoking, drinking, taking too much salty food, lack of daily exercise, and obesity. It is still possible for cerebral hemorrhage to occur in people who do not exhibit hypertension. This occurs when they have cerebral arteriovenous malformation, platelet disorder, or coagulation disorder.

It often suddenly develops during everyday working hours. The symptoms depend on the area of and the volume of the hemorrhage. The areas are mainly classified into the putamen, thalamus, brain stem, and cerebellum. In the case of putaminal hemorrhage, when the hematoma is big, the internal capsule is damaged, which causes hemiplegia. Whereas, when the damage occurs in the the dominant hemisphere, it may cause aphasia, when it is in the non-dominant hemisphere, it may cause apraxia and agnosia. In the case of thalamus hemorrhage, when the hematoma is big, the internal capsule is damaged and hemiplegia may occur but sensory disorder is rather serious and it may result in serious pain. In the case of brain stem hemorrhage, the patient quickly goes into coma, and it causes quadriplegia and myosis. It can rapidly result in sudden death: it has poor prognosis. In the case of cerebellar hemorrhage, there is no quadriplegia, but it causes ataxia, headache, nausea, emesis and dizziness.

For diagnosis, it is crucial to see the whole picture of symptoms, guess the hemorrhage area accurately, and make it sure with Head CT and MRI.

Within 24 hours of onset, there may be a danger of rebleeding, so it is important to start antihypertensive therapy in order to prevent rebleeding. As needed, drugs such as osmotic diuretics or steroids to reduce the symptoms of the intracranial hypertension. When brain herniation is evident, emergency craniotomy will be necessary. If there is any hematoma which has not be absorbed spontaneously, the blood mass removal operation should be performed after checking reduction of rebleeding risk and improvement of the brain edema is reduced.

That is the treatment during the acute phase of brain hemorrhage. If there is any deficit, rehabilitation will be the main treatment. If there is high blood pressure problem, antihypertensive therapy needs to be continued.

Brain hemorrhage is not as critical as subarachnoidal hemorrhage. It often has serious complications such as hemiplegia which is the major problem or speech disorder. So it leads to difficulty of social rehabilitation and necessity of everyday life.

Dialog at the clinic

クリニックでの対話

General practitioner (GP): Hello. What brings you here today, Ms Kawasaki?

Kawasaki (K): Hello, doc. I woke up with a terrible headache this morning and it's worse now. This is unusual for me.

GP: I see. Are you experiencing any other symptoms?

K: My vision is very blurred and my hands and fingers don't seem to work well.

GP: Are you feeling dizzy??

K: Yes, I feel very light headed when I stand up and the pain seems to get more intense.

GP: OK then, we are going to send you for MRI immediately so that we can rule out cerebral hemorrhage.

K: Oh dear.

GP: Don't panic, you'll be ok. You are in good hands here.

K: Ok, doc. I'll try to relax.

Exercise After reading the dialog, find answers to the following questions. 対話文を読んだあと，次の質問に答えなさい。

1. What caused Ms Kawasaki's headache?
2. What other symptoms did she have apart from a headache?
3. Why did the GP send her for MRI?

Grammar Review 原級, 比較級, 最上級

原級を使った比較の表現　形容詞や副詞の原級と as ... as
意味は「～と同じくらい～だ」「～ほど～ではない」となります。

A registered dietitian is as busy as a pharmacist at hospital.
管理栄養士は薬剤師と同じくらい病院で忙しい。

My brother is not as kind as my sister.
私の兄は姉ほど優しくない。

比較級を使った表現　形容詞や副詞の比較級＋than …
意味は「…より～だ」となります。

The doctor begins to work earlier than any other staff in this hospital.
あの医師はこの病院でどのスタッフよりも早く働き始める。

最上級を使った比較の表現　形容詞や副詞の最上級に the をつける
意味は「最も～だ」となります。

This department is the biggest in this hospital.

Exercise Underline the positive degree, the comparative degree and the superlative degree, and put each sentence into Japanese. 以下の文の原級，比較級，最上級にそれぞれ下線を引き，和訳しなさい。

1. This hospital is good, that one is better, but ours is the best.
2. This kidney is not as healthy as yours, but that one is the healthiest.
3. This surgeon is not as skillful as the resident, but your surgeon is the most skilled.
4. Your temperature is not as high as yesterday, but the day before it was the highest.
5. This painkiller is strong, that one is stronger, but morphine is the strongest.

Chapter 12

The Peripheral Nervous System

末梢神経系

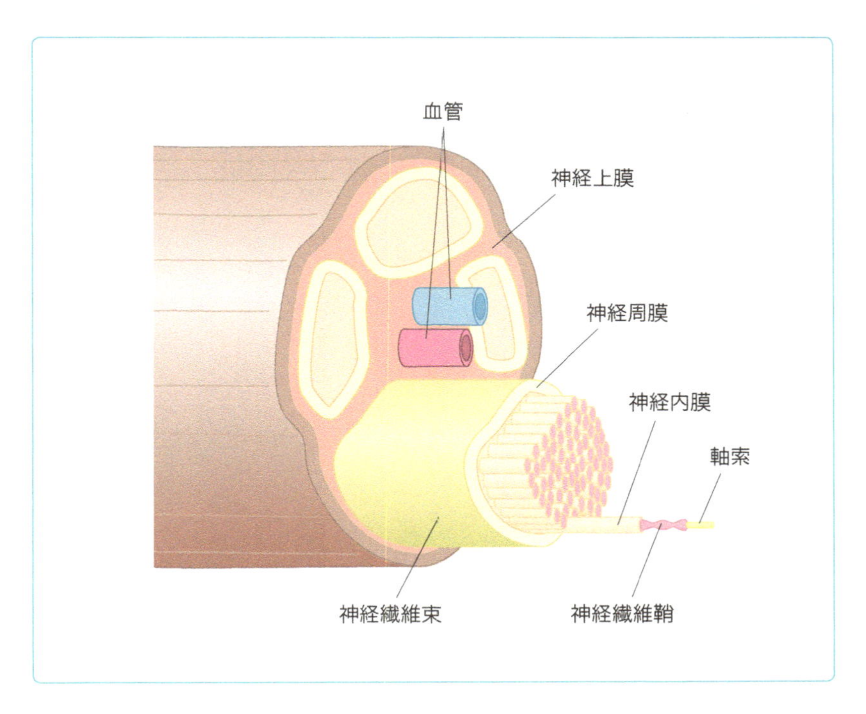

Objectives of this Chapter　本章の目的

Anatomy and physiology	Understanding the functions and the constituents of the peripheral nervous system 末梢神経系の機能と構造を理解する
Disease	Learning the pathology of the peripheral nervous system 末梢神経系の病理について学ぶ
Dialog	Talking about an operation and a peripheral nervous disorder 末梢神経疾患の手術に関する対話
Grammar review	Reviewing relative pronoun 関係代名詞について復習する

Anatomy and Physiology of the Peripheral Nervous System and Skin

末梢神経系と皮膚の解剖生理

Medical Terminology

afferent nerve	求心性神経
animal nervous system	動物神経系
autonomic nervous system	自律神経
cerebral nerves	脳神経
cervical nerves	頸神経
coccygeal nerve	尾骨神経
connective tissue	結合組織
cranial nerves	脳神経
dermatome	デルマトーム
dermis	真皮
efferent nerve	遠心性神経
epidermis	表皮
fatty layer	脂肪層
hypodermal tissue	皮下組織
lumber nerves	腰神経
median nerve	正中神経
Meissner's corpuscle	マイスナー小体
motor nervous system	運動神経系
neuralgia	神経痛
Pacinian corpuscle	パチニ小体
papillary layer	乳頭層
parasympathetic nervous system	副交感神経系
peripheral nervous system	末梢神経系
plexiform layer	網状層
plexus brachialis	腕神経叢
sacral nerves	仙骨神経
sensory nervous system	感覚神経系
sensory neurons	感覚神経
shoulder girdle	肩甲帯
skin groove	皮膚小溝
skin ridge	皮膚小陵
somatic nervous system	体性神経系
spinal cord	脊髄
spinal nerves	脊髄神経
surface mucosa	表面粘膜
sympathetic nervous system	交感神経系
thoracic nerves	胸神経
ulnar nerve	尺骨神経
vegetative nervous system	植物神経系
visceral tissue	内臓組織

Find answers to the following questions. 質問の答えを読み取ろう。

Q1. What is the CNS?

Q2. What is the PNS?

Q3. How does the motor nervous system work?

Q4. How does the autonomic nervous system work?

Q5. What is the largest organ in the body?

Q6. How is a fingerprint made?

The peripheral nervous system (PNS) comes out from the central nervous system (CNS) and spreads out throughout the whole body and reaches to the end of the body. The spinal cord is a meeting point of the brain and the PNS. The spinal cord has 31 segments, each with a pair of nerve roots equaling 31 spinal nerves. From the CNS to the PNS, there are 12 pairs of thoracic nerves, 8 pairs of cervical nerves, 5 pairs of lumber nerves, 5 pairs of sacral nerves, and 1 pair of coccygeal nerves. The nerves from the fifth cervical nerve to the eighth cervical nerve, and the first thoracic spinal nerve form a mesh like structure which is called the plexus brachialis, and this controls motion and perception from the scapular arch (shoulder girdle muscle) to the upper limbs. The PNS is generally divided into the somatic nervous system (SNS) (animal nervous system) and the autonomic nervous system (ANS) (plant nervous system). The former is further divided into the motor nervous system and the sensory nervous system. The motor nervous system is efferent nerves, which transmit from the CNS to the PNS, and they transmit signals from the CNS to the skeletal muscle in order to contract muscles and make joints move. On the other hand, the sensory nervous system are afferent nerves, which have the role of transmitting information from the PNS to the CNS, and they transmit various types of information from sensory organs, such as eyes, nose, skin, and so on to the central nerves. The autonomic nervous system is an autonomous neural mechanism, and communicates on surface mucosa of the smooth muscle, the myocardium, and the visceral tissue. The autonomic nervous system's afferent nerves are called visceral afferent nerves, which transmit sensations from internal organs such as pain. Moreover, the autonomic nervous system has a sympathetic nervous system and a parasympathetic nervous system, both having conflicting functions yet despite having an antagonistic effect, they work together.

If one peripheral nerve loses its function, which is called peripheral nerve paralysis, it makes the dominant muscle's contraction difficult, or causes sensory disorders in perception, which causes neuralgia in the dominant area.

The skin which covers the body is the largest organ, consisting of 6.3-6.9% of the weight. It is made of a top layer of surface skin, and under layer of inner skin. There is hypodermal tissue and various appendages such as hair, nails, and skin glands. The surface skin consists of 4-5 top layers, and the inner skin consists of connective tissue, both the papillary layer and the plexiform layer. The hypodermal tissue is mainly a fat layer. On the surface of the finger skin, there are lines which are called the skin ridges and the skin grooves, and they make finger prints when touched to a surface.

The main roles of the skin as a body surface organ are the protection of the inner organs against external hazards, maintaining body temperature, excreting waste such as perspiration, and skin respiration, and so on. Moreover, another important feature of the skin is to receive and send sensory stimulation. The body surface is a sensory organ having a sense of touch, pressure, pain, temperature, and so forth. This skin stimulus is delivered to the brain by the sensory receptors in the dermis called the Meissner's corpuscle and the Pacinian corpuscle.

A dermatome is an area of skin in which sensory nerves derive from a single spinal nerve root. The dermatome can be used to determine the location of origin of the skin’s sensory disorder. Diagnosis of peripheral nerve disorder, such as paralysis of the spiral nerve, median nerve, and ulnar nerve can be determined by locating the pain.

Disease Relevant to the Peripheral Nervous System

末梢神経系に関連する疾患

Medical Terminology

carpal tunnel syndrome	手根管症候群	motor function	運動機能
dorsiflexion	背屈	radial nerve paralysis	橈骨神経麻痺
elbow joint	肘関節	supracondylar fracture of humerus	上腕骨顆上骨
fracture of the humerus	上腕骨骨折	transverse carpal ligament	横手根靭帯
median nerve paralysis	正中神経麻痺	ulnar nerve paralysis	尺骨神経麻痺

Find answers to the following questions. 質問の答えを読み取ろう。

Q1. What is musculospiral paralysis?

Q2. What causes musculospinal paralysis?

Q3. What causes median nerve paralysis?

Q4. What is monkey hand?

Q5. What is claw hand?

Q6. What is ulnar nerve paralysis?

There are three major peripheral nervous disorders of the upper limbs: the radial nerve paralysis, median nerve paralysis, and ulnar nerve paralysis.

A) Radial nerve paralysis

Complication caused by compression of a nerve concurrently with the fracture of the humerus, by an injection to the upper arm, or by the pressure of the upper arm while sleeping. The radial nerve paralysis is, for the most part, impairment of the whole limb function caused by damage to the central nervous system. If there is damage to the peripheral nervous system, then individual muscles or a group of muscles in a specific location of the body are impaired.

The damage on the center part of the upper arm causes the dorsiflexion of the wrist joint, furthermore, it may become impossible to extend the MP joint and could cause a malformation called 'drop hand'. It could cause the sensory disorder of the thumb, the index finger, the dorsal side of the middle finger, and from the hand dorsal to the thumb side of the forearm.

B) Median nerve paralysis

Complication resulting from a supracondylar fracture and/or a wrist joint fracture, carpal tunnel syndrome could cause Median nerve paralysis.

Carpal tunnel syndrome is caused by strangulation of the median nerve of the carpal tunnel, which is made of the wrist bone and the ligamentum carpi transversum in the wrist joint. Impaired motor function in the hand causes the muscle of the thumb to atrophy, which causes thumb opposable disorder. This functional disorder is called monkey hand derived from the flattened hand resembling a monkey's paw not having an opposable thumb. The sensory disorder is observed from the thumb to half of the palm side of the fourth finger on the radial side.

C) Ulnar nerve paralysis

This complication results from damage to the ulnar nerve which runs from the shoulder to the little finger. It is associated with a fracture and/or incision wound of the cubital joint, or is caused by cubital tunnel syndrome.

Cubital tunnel syndrome is caused by chronic compression of the ulnar nerve at the cubital tunnel point which is composed of bones at the back of the medial epicondyle of the humerus and the ligament band.

As motor function becomes impaired by a contraction of interosseous muscles and hypothenar muscle, the fourth and fifth fingers' MP joints overextend and IP joint becomes crooked and deformed, due to muscle wasting. The muscle atrophy causes a deformity that makes the hand look like a claw known as claw hand. The sensory disorder is observed in the fifth and the fourth fingers, a half of the palm and dorsal side on the ulnar side.

Dialog about Peripheral nervous system

末梢神経系についての対話

A: What's up? Are you OK? You don't look well.

B: Well, I don't feel very well. In fact, I feel terrible.

A: What happened?

B: It looks like I should have an operation. I was diagnosed with "median nerve paralysis".

A: What? An operation!? How did it happen?

B: You know I had an accident a couple months ago.

A: Yes. When you were riding your bicycle, you were hit by a car, weren't you? But you said it was a minor injury at that time.

B: Yes. Although I didn't feel any pain, my right hand and thumb were damaged. So I became very clumsy, I mean I started dropping things, and the other day, I couldn't hold my granddaughter properly, so I nearly dropped her! Terrible!

A: Oh I'm sorry to hear that. But you had some treatment, didn't you?

B: Yes, physiotherapy and low frequent treatment. I thought it was getting better. But yesterday, my doctor said that the median nerve was damaged more than he thought and it may need surgery, nerve suture surgery.

A: Oh dear! But I remember my cousin had something like this done a few years ago. He said it was very quick and now he's glad he had it done.

B: Oh, I see. Thanks for telling me, I feel a little better hearing that.

Grammar Review 関係代名詞(relative pronoun)

関係代名詞　who, which, that

関係代名詞は文と文をつなぐ接続詞と代名詞の働きがあります。主節にある名詞（先行詞）を後ろから文が説明します。先行詞を修飾している文を形容詞節といいます。

（ex）

Nurses take care of my aunt kindly every day.

She suffers from chronic disease.

↓

Nurses take care of my aunt who suffers from chronic disease kindly every day.

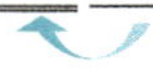

先行詞＼格	主格	所有格	目的格
人	who	whose	whom (who)
動物・事物	which	whose of which	which
人・動物・事物	that	–	that

Exercise　Underline the relative pronouns of the next sentences and translate into Japanese. 以下の文の関係代名詞に下線を引き，和訳しなさい。

1. We have just passed the old hospital which is closing.
2. This is the Renal Unit whose name was changed.
3. This is the kidney that you will be receiving.
4. We don’t know the person who donated the kidney.
5. He is the surgeon whom we would recommend.

Chapter 13

The Immune System

免疫系

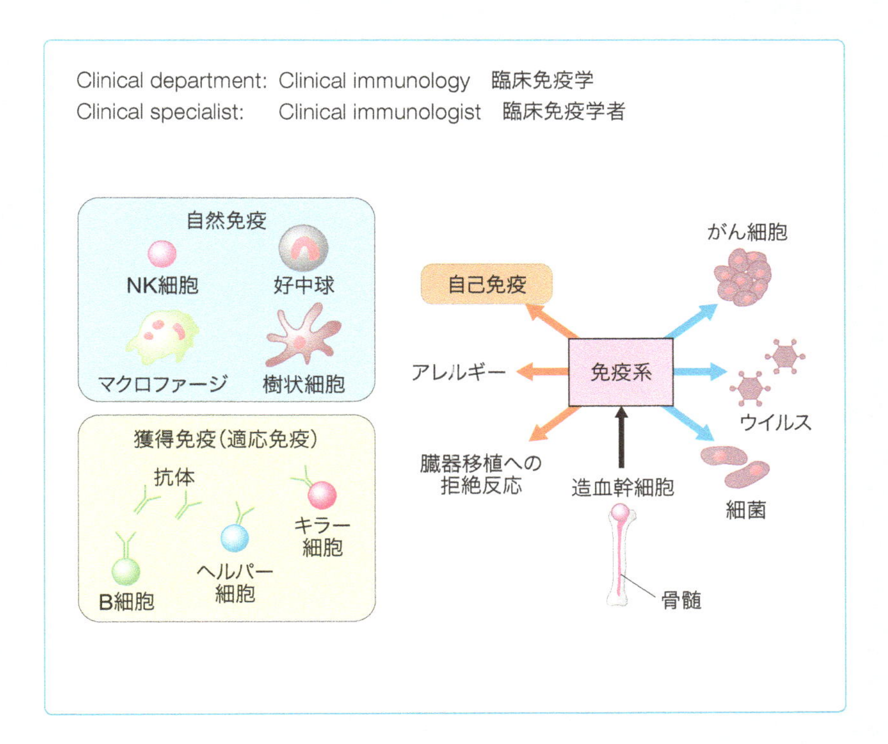

Objectives of this Chapter　本章の目的

Anatomy and physiology	Understanding the immune system 免疫系の理解
Disease	Learning about food poisoning　食中毒を学ぶ
Dialog	Discussing diarrhea　下痢について
Grammar review	Reviewing adjective usage of participles 分詞の形容詞用法について復習する

Anatomy and Physiology of the Immune System

免疫系の解剖生理

Medical Terminology

acquired immunity	獲得免疫
antibody	抗体
antigen presenting cells (【略】APCs)	抗原提示細胞
bacteria	細菌
chronic infection	慢性感染
defense mechanism	防御機構
dendritic cell	樹状細胞
enzyme	酵素
humoral immunity	液性免疫
infection	感染症
macrophage	マクロファージ
microbial antigen	微生物抗原
microorganism	微生物
monocyte	単球
natural immunity	自然免疫
neutrophil	好中球
penicillin	ペニシリン
phagocytic cell	食細胞
virus	ウイルス

Find answers to the following questions. 質問の答えを読み取ろう。

Q1. How does infection occur?

Q2. How does the body defend itself against microorganisms?

Q3. What are the two immune reactions when microorganisms enter the body?

Q4. What are phagocyte cells?

Q5. What is the difference between natural immunity and acquired immunity?

Q6. What happens to the immune response after the microorganism leaves the body?

Infection occurs when a microorganism invades the body, multiplies and migrates. These are microorganisms which can be identified as bacterial, viral, fungal or parasitic, bacterial and viral infections being the most common ones. It is true that there are good microorganisms which are beneficial for health as well. Although the number of microorganisms is vast, existing largely in the environment, there are only a few that can actually enter the host and cause disease. What can happen once a pathogen gains entry to the body?

Once the microorganism proliferate in the body, one of three things occurs:

1. The microorganism multiplies and destroys the body's protective immune system.
2. The microorganism achieves a state of balance and produces an acute or chronic infection.
3. The microorganism is destroyed by the immune response and eliminated from the body.

Microorganisms which cause disease seem to have a way of blocking the defense mechanism of the body and reinforcing the disease. For example, one of them produces an enzyme which destroys the body's immune system, and then it spreads infection rapidly over a wider area. Occasionally some microorganisms suddenly develop a method of blocking the immune defense mechanism, despite not having the ability earlier on. For example, a microorganism exposed to penicillin sometimes becomes resistant to penicillin due to rapid mutation of the pathogen. So, how does the human body fight against microorganisms?

Once the microorganism breaks through the body's first defense barrier, the skin or mucous membrane, two different immune reactions occur: natural immunity and acquired immunity. Natural immunity is an innate response to microorganisms, therefore, it needs no previous exposure to the microorganism beforehand. Even without immune memory, it reacts to foreign pathogens immediately. The natural immune cells include phagocytic cells, which also include the neutrophil, the monocyte and the macrophage, capture the foreign pathogens and destroy them fairly quickly. The natural killer cells kill virus-infected cells and parts of tumor cells as well. The neutrophil and monocyte destroy the microorganism and release the inflammatory mediators. On the other hand, acquired immunity takes more time before becoming activated, because it needs to be exposed to the microorganism beforehand, however, once it has been exposed, then it responds quite swiftly. The immune system conveniently memorizes this past exposure. There are two kinds of acquired immunities: humoral immunity known as antibodies coming from B-cells, and cellular immunity derived from T-cells. B-cells and T-cells work together to destroy foreign substances, and during this process, antigen presentation cells called dendritic cells need to show the microbial antigen to the T-cells. Activation of the immune response, known as adjustment, can succeed in immune defense. When the circulating antibody or the receptor on the surface of the cell recognizes the microorganism, it activates itself. If the T-cell properly adjusts, then it blocks immune reaction to the host. When the microorganism is finally flushed out of the body, the immune response disappears.

Useful information 免疫力って？

免疫力が下がると，「なんとなくだるい，体調を崩しやすい，風邪を引きやすい，肌荒れがひどくなる」などといわれますね。さらに体温が下がると免疫力も下がることがわかっています。近年の研究で，マウスを20℃，4℃，−12℃に置いて免疫に関連する細胞数を数えた結果，寒いほど免疫を抑制する細胞が減り，自己免疫疾患を引き起こすかもしれないという結論が出ています。色々な免疫力アップ方法，運動，睡眠，つぼ押し，呼吸法，食事等がありますが，やはり食生活が一番大事ですね！　体を冷やさず，体温を上げる食事が重要です。季節の食材，体を温める食材を使いましょう。氷は厳禁です。次の食材は体を温めます。体を温めて免疫力をアップしましょう！

体を温める食材：酢，りんご，ローヤルゼリー，ヨモギ，うなぎ，マグロ，牡蠣，にら，生姜，落花生，ねぎ，しそ，コショウ，らっきょ，山椒，納豆，味噌，など。

Food poisoning

食中毒

Medical Terminology

anisakis	アニサキス	infant botulism	乳児ボツリヌス症
campylobacter	カンピロバクター	laryngitis	喉頭炎
diarrhea	下痢	norovirus	ノロウイルス
enterohemorrhagic *Escherichia coli*	腸管出血性大腸菌	parasite	寄生虫
gastrointestinal symptom	胃腸症状	*salmonella*	サルモネラ菌

Find answer to the following questions. 質問の答えを読み取ろう。

Q1. What is infant botulism?

Q2. What are the causes of food poisoning?

Q3. What was the tragic incident of the 6- month-old infant?

Q4. What are the symptoms of food poisoning?

Q5. Why can't botulism survive in the bodies of adults?

Food poisoning is a serious illness caused by eating contaminated food. Contamination can occur through growing, harvesting, processing, storing or shipping or even in food preparation. Infectious organisms such as bacteria, virus, parasite, natural plant poison, and/or the toxins they produce are the most common causes of food contamination. Once contaminated food is consumed and has time to incubate, within hours, gastrointestinal symptoms including nausea, diarrhea, fever and/or vomiting appear. Symptoms can last from a few hours to several days.

Food poisoning happens all year round, however, bacterial poisoning occurs, most often in summer. The major microbes causing illnesses are enterhemorrhagic *Escherichia coli* (for example O157 *E.coli*), *campylobacter*, and *salmonella*. On the other hand, microbes which survive in cold temperatures or in dry climates, such as the norovirus, cause illness in winter, spreading rapidly via food handling of raw, ready to eat produce and fish from contaminated water in restaurants, school cafeterias, etc.. . This seems to count for over 50% of reported food poisoning cases. Apart from that, the parasite such as anisakis carried by mackerel, horse mackerel, and octopus could cause food poisoning

Sixty percent of food poisoning happens in restaurants, but also occurs in nursing homes, at social functions, and in school cafeterias. Only 10% seems to happen at home through improper storage, washing, cooking of food, and from expired dairy, meat, or fish products.

Treatments depend on the source of the poisoning and on the severity of the symptoms. Bacterial infections may require antibiotics, however, the doctor will determine the course of treatment after assessment. Most times bed rest and fluids are recommended. To prevent dehydration, sucking on ice chips or taking small sips of water is beneficial. Avoid eating too soon, drink soup and/or consume soft foods such as bananas, soft rice or soda crackers. and of course, get plenty of rest.

After the report of the tragic death of a 6-month-old infant who was fed honey as baby food, and as a result, suffered from infant botulism, the ministry of Health and Labor and Welfare stated: "Give your baby honey only after the first year birthday". The botulinus is always there, and sometimes is present in honey. For adults, the botulinus can't survive after fighting with other bacteria in the intestine, however, in the case of infants, the botulinus may predominate and produce poison (toxin) in the intestine of infants because of immature intestinal environment.

In order to prevent infant botulism, avoid giving under-one-year old infant food such as honey, food or drink containing honey, which may be contaminated by the botulism spore which could strongly resist heat, medicine, dryness, and hibernate for a long time, waiting for the right environment to spread.

Dialog about Diarrhea

下痢についての対話

Medical Terminology

diarrhea	下痢	rehydration	水分補給
laryngitis	喉頭炎	Salmonella	サルモネラ菌
pulse	脈	throat lozenges	喉あめ

Tom (T): Hi, how was your trip to India?

John (J): Well, sadly, I spent most of the time in the hotel bathroom.

T: Oh dear! What happened?

J: I got food poisoning on the first day. I had terrible diarrhea and a fever. I felt so bad and so the hotel staff called a doctor.

T: And then?

J: He checked my pulse, temperature and blood. He prescribed re-hydration salts in the meantime.

T: Rehydration salts?

J: Yes, apparently this treatment works for diarrhea.

T: Did you find out the cause?

J: It turned out to be some form of Salmonella. It took me a whole week before I could eat again.

T: Oh, nasty business! Speaking of which, my friend lost her voice coming back from holiday.

J: Oh, what caused that?

T: The doctor thinks it's laryngitis, she possibly picked it up from the plane ride.

J: Laryngitis? Did he give her antibiotics?

T: No, laryngitis is not a bacterial infection, it is a viral infection.

J: Oh I didn't know that. Is she better now?

T: Yes, it didn't last for too long. She was given throat lozenges and used a hot wet towel periodically around her neck.

Grammar Review 分詞の形容詞用法

分詞には現在分詞と過去分詞の2種類があります。名詞用法，形容詞用法，副詞用法があり，分詞が名詞を修飾するのが形容詞用法です。

現在分詞　動詞の原形＋ing「〜している」「〜する」の意味で名詞を修飾する。
過去分詞　「〜されている」「〜された」の意味で名詞を修飾する。

＊分詞＋名詞　分詞だけの時は名詞の前に置く。

a broken window　　a crying baby

＊名詞＋分詞　分詞が他の語句と一緒の時は名詞の後に置く（分詞の後置修飾）。

a baby crying over there　　a window broken by Tom

Exercise　Change a verb in (　) to its proper grammatical form.（　）内の動詞を適切な形に変えなさい。

1. These are more than 50 % of the (treat) patients.
2. There is a (sleep) baby in the intensive care unit.
3. An (injure) man is waiting for a bed.
4. His (broke) arm should be reset immediately.
5. I know the girl (sit) by the window.
6. Is that the bag (send) to you by your mother?
7. My friend can read books (write) in Chinese easily.
8. The nurses (take) care of old people are very kind.

英文索引

和文索引

あ行

か行

さ行

た行

な行

は行

ま行

や ら行

編著者紹介

髙木久代(たかぎひさよ)　鈴鹿医療科学大学保健衛生学部教授

NDC490　111p　21cm

やさしいメディカル英語(えいご)

2018年6月29日　第1刷発行
2020年2月20日　第2刷発行

編著者　髙木久代(たかぎひさよ)
発行者　渡瀬昌彦
発行所　株式会社 講談社
〒112-8001　東京都文京区音羽2-12-21
販　売　(03) 5395-4415
業　務　(03) 5395-3615

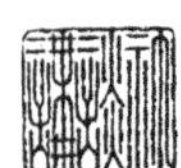

編　集　株式会社 講談社サイエンティフィク
代表　矢吹俊吉
〒162-0825　東京都新宿区神楽坂2-14　ノービィビル
編　集　(03) 3235-3701

本文データ制作　株式会社 エヌ・オフィス
カバー・表紙印刷　豊国印刷 株式会社
本文印刷・製本　株式会社 講談社

落丁本・乱丁本は，購入書店名を明記のうえ，講談社業務宛にお送りください。送料小社負担にてお取替えいたします。なお，この本の内容についてのお問い合わせは，講談社サイエンティフィク宛にお願いいたします。定価はカバーに表示してあります。

Printed in Japan

ISBN 978-4-06-511935-8